PATTY—BRIDE

Patty – Bride

BY

CAROLYN WELLS

Author of
The TWO LITTLE WOMEN *Series*
The MARJORIE *Books*
etc.

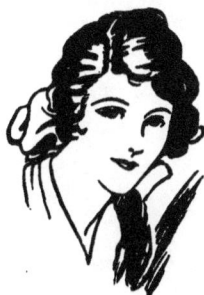

GROSSET & DUNLAP, *Publishers*
NEW YORK

CONTENTS

Patty-Bride

CHAPTER I

PHILIP'S CHANCE

"I CAN'T *stand* it, Patty, I simply *can't* stand it!"

"But you'll have to, Phil, dear. I'm engaged to Little Billee, and some day I'm going to marry him. And that's all there is about it."

"Oh, no, Patty, that isn't all about it. I'm not going to give you up so easily. You don't *know* how I care for you. You've no idea what a determined chap I can be,——"

"Now, stop, Phil. You know you promised that we should be friends and nothing more. You promised not to ask for more than my friendship—didn't you, now?"

"I did but that was only so you'd stay friendly with me, and I thought,—forgive the egotism,—I thought I could yet win your love.

[9]

Patty, you don't care such a lot for Farnsworth, do you, now?"

"Indeed I do, Phil. Why, do you suppose
I'd be engaged to him if I didn't love him more
than anybody in all the world? Of course I
wouldn't!"

"I know you think so, Patty," Phil's handsome face was grave and kind, "but you may
be mistaken."

"I'm not mistaken, Philip, and unless you
change your subject of conversation, I'll have
to ask you to go away. I should think you'd
scorn to talk like that to a girl who's engaged
to another man!"

"I should think I would, too, Patty. But I
can't help it. Oh, my girl, my little love, I
can't give you up. I can't tamely stand aside
and make no effort to win you back! I'm not
asking anything wrong, Patty, only don't send
me away; let me try once again for you,——"

"It's too late, Phil," and Patty looked a little frightened at his vehemence.

"It's never too late, until you're actually
married to him. When will that be?"

"Oh, I don't know. We've only been engaged a fortnight,——"

"And I only learned of it today,——"

"I know, I tried to get you on the tele-phone,——"

"Yes, I've been down in Washington for a week or more. But, Patty, dearest, think how surprised and stunned I was to hear of it. I came right over, to learn from you, yourself, if it could be true."

"Yes, Philip, it is true, and I'm glad and happy about it. I'm sorry you've been disap-pointed, but—there are others——"

"Hush!" and Van Reypen fairly glared at her, "never imply that there's any one else in the world for me! Oh, Patty, my little Patty, I can't bear it."

His great, dark eyes were full of despair, his face was drawn with sorrow, and Patty for-gave him, even while she resented his atti-tude.

"You mustn't, Philip," she said, gently; "it isn't right for you to talk to me like that. I feel disloyal, even to listen to it."

"I don't care!" Van Reypen burst out. "You're mine! You promised Aunty Van you'd marry me! You *promised!*"

Philip grasped her hand in both his own, and gazed at her so wildly that Patty was tempted to run out of the room. But she realised the

[11]

matter must be settled once for all, and she spoke with dignity.

"Philip," she said, "I don't think you're quite fair to me,—or to Billee. Is it manly to talk like this to the girl who is promised to your friend?"

"No, it isn't. You're right, Patty." Van Reypen dropped her hand and folding his arms, stood and looked at her. "But listen to me, girl. I shall not give up until you're married to Farnsworth. If I can win you back from him, I'm going to do so. I shall do nothing wrong. But, dear, I'm so miserable,—so utterly heart-broken,—you won't put me out of your life,—will you?"

Now one of Patty's strongest traits of character was her dislike of giving pain to another. Philip could have put forth no more powerful argument than an avowal of his disappointment. Against her better judgment, even against her own wish, she smiled kindly on him.

"I don't want to put you out of my life, Phil, but I can't let you talk to me like this,——"

"I won't, Patty. Just let me see you once in a while, let me keep on loving you, and then, if

you really love Bill better than you do me, I'll
see it,—I'll know it, and I'll give you up."

"All right, then, but you must promise not
to tell me you care for me."

Van Reypen gave a short, hard laugh. "Not
tell you! When I don't tell you, I won't be
breathing! Why, Patty, I can't any more help
telling you, than I can help loving you. But I
promise not to make your life a burden,—or
myself a nuisance. Trust me, dear. I don't
mean to steal you away from Bill,—unless you
want to be stolen."

"I don't!" and Patty's smile and blush
showed plainly where her heart had been
given.

Phil winced, but he said, blithely, "Very good,
my lady. There's no use being too down-
hearted about it all. Give me my chance,—
that's all I ask."

"But, Phil, the time for your ' chance ' as you
call it, is past. I'm engaged to Little Billee;—
to me that's as sacred, as unbreakable a promise, as my marriage vows will be."

"Oh, no, it isn't! Lots of people break off
an engagement."

Philip's lightness annoyed Patty, and her
mood changed.

" Well, then," she said, " if you can so bewitch me that I *want* to break my engagement to Bill Farnsworth, I'll do it, but you've about as much chance as—as nothing at all ! "

" I'll *make* a chance ! Oh, Patty, don't forget you said that ! Don't forget you said if I can win you away from him, I may do so ! Listen, dear. I'm not over conceited, or vain, but I do think that you don't quite know your own mind, and you're a little bit dazzled by Bill's big masterfulness and you don't realise that perhaps there are other things worth while."

" I don't know what you're talking about, but I'll stick to my word. And I'll add that I know you *never* can cut Bill out, because I love him too much. So, there now ! "

" Maybe I can't, maybe you're right, but I'll have a go at it, all the same."

" Of course, you know, I'll tell him of this conversation."

" Of course you may. There's nothing underhanded about my determination. If I can win you from him, it'll be done fairly, and in that case, Bill's own sense of justice would make him willing to give you up."

" Little Billee give me up !   Willingly? *Nevaire!* "

Philip's Chance

"He would, Patty, if you told him yourself that you loved me more."

"Oh, *that!* But I've no expectation of ever doing that."

"Who can say? You're a fickle little thing, you know——"

"Indeed I'm not!"

"Yes, you are, and always have been. You're fond of Bill just now, because he's been doing the caveman act, carrying you off from the Blaney party, and such things, but you'll soon tire of him,——"

"Stop, Philip! I won't listen to such talk."

Patty put her hands over her ears and pouted. It was nearing twilight of an afternoon in late January, and the two were in the library of the Fairfield home. Patty had become engaged to Farnsworth while on a visit to Adele Kenerley, and had but lately returned from there.

This was her first interview with Philip since her engagement, and she had dreaded it, for she knew Phil's stubborn and persistent nature would not tamely submit to an end of his hopes. Patty had firmly resolved that if Philip insisted on telling her of his love for her, she would refuse to see him at all; but her gentle heart could not let her summarily dismiss him. She temporised, not because she cared for him, or had the least thought of disloyalty to Farnsworth, but because she couldn't bear to hurt him by forbidding him to come to her home.

She tried to change the subject. She was sitting in the corner of a huge davenport, and her little house dress of pink Georgette was very becoming. She rather hoped that Farnsworth would come in while Phil was there, but it was uncertain whether he could arrive before dinner or not until evening.

"I won't listen," she repeated; "if you'll talk about something else, nod your head, and I'll stay; but if not, shake your head, and I'll run off to my own room."

Van Reypen nodded his head, and Patty took her hands away from her ears.

"All right," she said, smiling; "if you'll be just a casual friend, go ahead and be it. But I don't want to hear any more absurd talk about people's breaking their engagements."

"Righto! What shall we talk about?"

"About Bill."

This might have proved a dangerous subject, but clever Philip would not allow it to be. He was honest and earnest in his love for Patty. He really believed that she had said yes to

Philip's Chance

Farnsworth on the spur of the moment, and that further thought would make her willing to reconsider her decision. Moreover, he was quite willing his rival should know of his own intentions, and he had only feelings of good fellowship for him. Philip had a sportsman's nature, and his idea was to let the best man win. He did not attach quite so much importance to the fact of the engagement as most people do, and he truly hoped yet to win Patty's affection and make her both willing and anxious to dismiss Bill in his favour.

Patty had not given him any encouragement for these hopes. In fact, she was so truly in love with Farnsworth, that it never occurred to her that she could ever care less for him, or have any room in her heart for any other man. But she couldn't seem to say this bluntly to Philip. She found it easier to let matters drift, and now, as he began to speak in praise of Farnsworth, she listened eagerly and assented and agreed to all Philip said.

"Yes, he is splendid," she acquiesced. "I didn't know there was such a noble nature in the world. You see, I've learned a lot about him since we've been engaged."

"Oh, of course. Yes, old Bill is a corker for

bigness in every way. I'm banking on his big nature and his broad outlook, to understand my case."

"Now, now, you're not to talk of 'your case'! You promised not to."

"With thee conversing, I forget all—promises!" misquoted Philip.

"Well, you mustn't, or I'll send you packing! Thank goodness, here comes Nan; *now* will you behave yourself?"

Mrs. Fairfield came in from out-of-doors, and drew near the blazing log fire.

"Well, children, what are you discussing so seriously?" she began; "Philip, my friend, if you please, will you push that bell and let us have lights and some tea. I've been to three committee meetings and I'm just about exhausted. Where's Billee-boy, Patty?"

"I'm afraid he won't be here until after dinner. He said it was unlikely he could come before."

"Well, try to bear it, Patty. Can't Philip beguile you for a time?"

"Yes, he's a great little old beguiler, Phil is!" and Patty smiled at her guest.

"Of course I am," declared Van Reypen. "I can beguile the birds off the trees,—but *not*

Philip's Chance

Miss Patricia Fairfield, when she is waiting for her big Little Billee. Howsumever, I'll do my best. Do I gather that I'm asked to dinner in place of the absentee?"

"You are *not!*" replied Patty, promptly, but Nan said, "Why, yes, Phil, stay. I'll entertain you, if Patty won't."

"Thank you, Ma'am. That would suit me all right."

"And how about your aviation training? When do you begin that?"

"It's uncertain. I did expect to start for Wilmington next week, but matters are delayed by a screw loose in some of the red tape, and it may be a couple of weeks before I start."

"What? I didn't know you thought of going," put in Patty, surprised.

"Yes, I've settled the preliminaries and I'm waiting further orders."

"Going to Wilmington? Why, we won't see you any more, then."

"You don't seem terribly upset over that! But, you will see me, I'm afraid. Wilmington is not so very far off, and the course is neither long nor strenuous. Why, it only takes about four months in all."

"And then will you really fly? Up in the air, in big machines?"

"Such is my firm belief, Mademoiselle."

"And will you fall and break your neck? They say they all do."

"I'll not promise to do that, unless you insist upon it. And it isn't done as much as formerly, I believe."

"Why are you two sparring so?" asked Nan, laughingly. "Aren't you good friends, at the moment?"

"As good as anybody can be, when the lady he admires has been and went and gone and engaged herself to somebody else," and Philip frowned darkly.

"Oho, so that's it! Well, our young friend here is certainly engaged to her big Western suitor. Now, shall I look out for a sweet little girl for you?"

"No, thank you, Ma'am, it's a case of Patty or nobody, where I'm concerned. But the game's never out till it's played out. Patty and Farnsworth may one or both of them yet change their minds."

"You wouldn't think so, if you saw them together," laughed Nan. "They're just about the most engagedest pair you ever saw!"

"Oh, come now," said Patty, "we don't show our affection in public, Nan!"

"Well, you have great difficulty not to do so. It's all you can do, to hide it successfully."

"And why should they?" asked Phil. "There's no law against that sort of thing, is there?"

"Tell me more about your aviating," said Patty, by way of changing the subject. "What do you do to learn?"

"Dunno myself, yet. They say the only way to learn to swim is to be thrown into the water. So I daresay the way to learn to fly, is to get in an aeroplane and start."

"Nonsense! You have to be taught."

"Then I will be taught. But I'm going to be a good aviator. I'm sure I'll like the stunt, and I want to begin as soon as possible."

"I wish I could do some war work," and Patty sighed.

"Good gracious!" said Nan, "I don't know any girl who does more of it than you do, Patty! When you're not down in that old office doing clerical work, you're knitting like a house afire. And you are on two or three committees and you write slogans for the Food people and for the Liberty Loan Bonds, and oh, I don't know what all you do!"

"All of a sudden, isn't it?" asked Philip, interestedly. "Have you been doing these things long?"

"Some of them," said Patty. "But I have done more of late. I feel so useless unless I do."

"Yes," said Nan, "and then you work beyond your strength, and overtax yourself, and the first thing you know you will be useless indeed!"

"Why, Patty? Why these great works?" asked Van Reypen.

"Oh, because of Bill," Nan answered for her. "You see he's so mixed up in war work, that Patty must needs to do a lot also. And she's such an extremist, she's not satisfied with doing a *bit*, it must be a whole lot of bits."

"Don't believe her, Phil," said Patty, gaily. "I do what I can, and no more. Also, I'm going to put a stop to this idea that I'm a delicate plant,—for I'm not. I'm as healthy as— as a backwoodsman."

"Fine comparison. Your sturdiness is exactly that of a backwoodsman! You could haul logs, if you want to, I dare say."

"Don't be funny. But I am heaps stronger than I used to be. It's a whole lot better for me to *do* things than to sit around and be coddled."

"That's true, Patty. What are you doing, that I can help you with? Any sort of work where you could use a pair of willing hands?"

"But you're going off aviating——"

"Haven't gone yet! Dunno when I will go. In the mean time let me help you. What's your newest plan?"

"Well, for one thing, I'm going to help entertain the boys in khaki. A committee has asked me to, and if Nan agrees, I mean to devote one evening a week to it. Say we ask a few to dinner, and some more to come in the evening, and have some music and games and make it pleasant for them."

"Count me in. I'll gladly help out with such a program. Even after I go to Wilmington, I can get up here once a fortnight at least,— maybe, oftener."

"All right. Now, what I'm thinking out, is how to make it pleasant for the boys we invite. I'd like to give them some real pleasure, not only some music and silly chatter."

" Such as what? I mean, what have you in mind? "

" Well, I thought of getting some interesting lecturer——"

" Cut it out, Patty. They don't want lectures, —of all things! '

" What do they want? "

" I think the most of them want just a home atmosphere, and a few hours of pleasant company, without much reference in the chat to war conditions."

" Do you think so? "

" I'm sure of it. If you ask half a dozen soldiers and have your father and Mrs. Fairfield here, and a few girl friends of yours, if you like, I'll guarantee your visitors will be better entertained than if you had the finest lecturer that ever droned out a lot of platitudes."

" All right, Philip, you help me to get up such a party, and try it,—will you? "

" I sure will, and that with much quickness. Shall we say a week from tonight? "

" Yes that will be fine. I'll ask Elise and——"

" Don't go too fast. I'll find the khaki boys first, and then you get the rest."

" All right," agreed Patty.

CHAPTER II

BUMBLE ARRIVES

"HELLO! Patty Popinjay! Where are you?"

As a matter of fact, Patty was curled up in a big armchair near the library fire, waiting for that very voice.

"Here I am!" she cried in return and jumped up to be grabbed in the arms of a handsome, jolly-looking girl who came flying into the room. "Oh, Bumble, I'm so glad to see you!"

The newcomer laughed.

"Bumble!" she exclaimed; "I haven't heard that name for years. Let me look at you, Patty. My! you're prettier than ever! Well, I just *had* to come. I couldn't resist, when I heard of your engagement. Where's the man? Show him to me at once!"

"Oh, he isn't here, for the moment. But you'll see him soon. I'm only afraid you'll cut me out. Why, Bumble,—Helen, I mean, you're utterly changed from the little girl I remember."

"Of course I am—in appearance,—but no other way."

"Are you still the happy-go-lucky, hit-or-miss little rascal you used to be?"

"Of course I am. Oh, Patty, doesn't it seem long ago that you spent that summer with us? And to think I've scarcely seen you since! Not since Nan's wedding, anyway."

"No; and you only in Philadelphia! It's ridiculous. But, I've tried to get you over here time and again."

"I know it. But I went out West to Stanford, and I was there so long, I almost lost track of all my Eastern people. Your Best Beloved is Western, isn't he? Oh, Patty, tell me all,—everything about him."

"All in good time, Helen, honey. For now, I'll just say that he's the dearest and best man in the whole world, and that you'll agree to that when you see him. Now, come up to your room, and fix yourself up. You look as if you'd been through a whirlwind!"

"I always look like that," and Helen Barlow laughed.

Bumble Arrives

She was Patty's cousin, and had come to New York for a visit. She had often been invited and several times had planned to come, but something had prevented her, and as the Barlow family were of a most undependable sort in the matter of keeping engagements or appointments, it surprised nobody that Helen had not carried out her plans. Indeed the surprise was that she was really here at last, and Patty stared at her hard to reassure herself that her guest had positively appeared.

Helen Barlow was a pretty girl, about Patty's own age. Her soft brown hair was curled round her ears, in the prevailing mode, but it showed various wisps out of place, and needed certain pats and adjustments before a mirror. Her hat, a brown velvet toque, was a little askew,—even more so than she meant it to be, —and the long fur stole, over her arm, dragged on the floor.

Without being positively unkempt, Helen was untidy, and Patty well remembered that as a child she had been far more so.

The two girls went up to the room prepared for Helen, and soon her outer garments went flying. The hat was tossed on the bed, upside down; the stole slipped to the floor as the long

[27]

cloth coat was wrenched open and one button pulled off by an impatient twitch.

" Never mind," Helen said, " that old button was loose, anyway. Oh, Patty, how trim and tidy *you* look! "

It was second nature to Patty to be well groomed, and she would have been sadly uncomfortable with a button missing or a ribbon awry, unless intentionally so. For Patty was no prim young person, but she was by no means untidy.

She laughed at her cousin's impetuous ways, and picked up the scattered garments, as fast as Helen flung them down.

" Don't you have a maid, Patty? I supposed of course you did."

" Oh, we have Jane. She maids Nan and me both, when we want her. But she does a lot of other things, too. We don't have as many servants as we used to. Patriotism has struck this house, you know, and we've cut out more or less of the luxuries."

" Good for you! I'm patriotic, too. Do you knit? "

" Of course; who doesn't? Now, Bumble,— oh, yes, I'm going to call you by the old name if I want to,—do try to make yourself look tidy! Take down your hair and do it over. Your hair is lovely,—if you'd take a little more pains with it."

" To be sure! Anything to please!" and Helen shook down her short curly mop. " Let me see his picture," she demanded as she brushed vigorously away. " Quick! quick! I can't wait a minute!"

Patty ran out of the room, laughing, and returned with a photograph of Farnsworth.

"Stunning!" cried Helen, " he's simply great! Wherever did you catch him? Are there any more at home like him? 'Deed I *will* steal him away from you, if I possibly can. Oh, Patty, do you remember Chester Wilde? Well, he wants me to marry him, but I can't see it! That's one reason I ran away from home, to escape his persistence."

" I do believe you're a belle, Bumble! You're fascinating, I see. Mercy goodness, you'll cut poor little me out with everybody!"

" As if you cared! Now that you're wooed and won!"

" Of course I don't care. You can have all the others,—and there are plenty,—only, so many of them are going or gone to war."

" I know, all my best ones have, too. But

[29]

you couldn't like a man who doesn't *want* to
fight!"

"I should say *nixie!*"

"What's your Bill do? Is he in camp?"

"Oh, no. You know, he's an expert mining
engineer, and he's used,—I mean, his services
are used by the government. I can't tell you
all about it, because I don't know all myself;
and what I do know, I'm not allowed to tell,
in detail. So don't ask, Helen; just know my
little Billee is doing his full duty,—and then
some!"

"Little! *Is* he little? He doesn't look so,
from this picture."

The photograph showed only the head and
shoulders of Farnsworth, but it hinted a large
man. However, Patty said, just for fun:

"You can't tell from that. But I don't
mind how little he is,—he's all the world to
me!"

She looked a trifle embarrassed, so, thinking
Farnsworth must be decidedly undersized,
Helen dropped the subject.

Her trunk had arrived, and Jane appeared, to
assist in unpacking.

"Get out a pretty frock," Patty directed her
guest, "and I'll help you get into it, and then

we'll go down and see Nan, she'll soon be home."

" Where is she? "

" Chasing some committee, as usual. We've both lost our individuality now, and we're merged in committees. I'm a member of quite a number, but Nan belongs to more than I do. Here, Helen, put on this bluet, Georgette, satinet thing."

" Rather dressy? "

" Not too much so. It's nearly tea time, and people often drop in and I want you to make a good impression. And for gracious' sake, do your hair more carefully than that! Here, let me do it,—or Jane."

" All right," and Helen dropped into a chair before the toilette table, while the deft and willing Jane quickly twisted up the brown locks.

" Now you'll do," said Patty, after a final critical examination. " Oh, wait, this sash end is loose."

" I know, the snapper's off. Never mind."

" But I do mind! Helen Barlow, you're as bumbly as ever! We used to call you that because you were as heedless and careless as a bumblebee——"

"There was another reason," Helen laughed.

"Yes, because you were so fat! You've pretty nearly gotten over that."

"Thank you, lady, for dem kind woids! A little guarded, aren't you? Know then, that my sole end, aim and ambition is to get thin, really thin,—slim, slender, willowy,—merely a slip of a girl——"

"You haven't quite achieved all that!" and Patty laughed. "But if you're trying to, I'll help you. No sweets, you know."

"Gracious, Patty, I haven't tasted candy for two years! And as a sugar conserver, I'm right there! Not a lump of it comes *my* way!"

"Good for you! Then, with exercise, and not too much sleep, we'll soon get you into condition!"

The girls went down stairs, and found Nan already there.

"My dear old Bumble!" she cried; "no, no Helen for me! I knew you too long by the old name to change."

"But, Nan, I don't like it! Please don't. Such a horrid name!"

"All right, then. I'll try to say Helen, but if the other slips out sometimes, you must for-

[32]

give me.   Now, how's everybody?   Bob all right?"

"Fine!   In camp, of course, but he gets home occasionally, or we go to see him.   Dad and Mother sent all sorts of messages and greetings,—and hoped I won't make you too much trouble—as if I *could!*"

"Indeed you can't!" cried Nan, warmly. "We're just awfully glad to see you, and you must stay just as long as you possibly can. Has Patty been telling you of her latest escapade?"

"She wrote me of it,—that's mostly why I came.   I thought the sight of the flirtatious, coquettish, altogether frivolous and fickle Patty Fairfield tied down to one man, would be worth seeing!"

"Huh!" remarked Patty, "when you see the man, you'll not wonder!   Anybody would be glad to be tied to him."

"I'm going to cut Patty out, you know, Nan," Helen declared, "but it's more likely she'll throw him over and fly to some newer flame,——"

"Oh, *very* likely," Patty mocked, her eyes dancing, "oh, ve-*ry* like-*ly!*   When I throw him over, Bumble, you have my full permission to pick him up.   But until then,—hands off my property! "

The tea things appeared then, and Patty did the honours, remarking, " Yes, we do have tea, 'most every day, and we have sugar in it,—but we skimp it some and we don't have really rich cakes."

" I'm glad to get it," and Helen accepted her cup. " I forgot to get any luncheon, and I'll just make up for it now."

Whereupon she proceeded to devour cakes and biscuits, until Patty silently despaired of ever helping her in a quest for slimness!

But Patty looked at her cousin affectionately. Helen was so jolly and gay-looking, so wholesome and smiling, and so sincerely glad to be with them, that she made herself thoroughly welcome. Her dark eyes were beaming with good nature, her round, plump face was alight with good will and her laughter bubbled forth like a child's.

She put her little fat hand up to her lips. " Honest, I'm trying not to giggle so much," she said, " but I just can't help it! When I'm happy, I have to chuckle, and that's all about it."

" Giggle all you like, my dear," said Nan,

"I'm glad to hear it. There's so much sadness in the world, that a truly merry laugh like yours is infectious and does us all good. Now, make yourself at home, Helen, and don't mind it if I seem to neglect you. I'm not really going to do that, but I do have an awful lot to see to,——"

"Oh, I know, Nan. And Patty has, too. But I'll be a help, not a nuisance,—you see if I'm not. Why, Patty Fairfield! you said he was little!"

The original of the photograph she had seen, strode into the room and when Helen saw big Bill Farnsworth, she knew Patty had chaffed her.

Farnsworth went to Patty and grasped both her hands in his.

"All right?" he said, looking deep into her blue eyes.

"All right," Patty returned, with an answering gaze, and so true was the sympathy between them, that a sort of telepathic message was exchanged and further words were unnecessary.

Then Farnsworth turned to greet Nan, and to be presented to Miss Helen Barlow.

"She told me you were little!" Helen exclaimed, looking at the broad-shouldered giant who faced her.

"Not quite that, I think," Bill smiled at her, "Patty probably called me Little Billee, which is her pet name for her lord and master!"

"Future lord and master!" corrected Patty, "not yet, not yet, my child!"

"'Serene I fold my hands, and wait,'" Farnsworth quoted, with undisturbed equanimity. "I'm very glad you've come, Miss Barlow. Perhaps you can entertain Patty and keep her from getting *too* impatient at the time that must elapse before I can take her for keeps."

"Vanity Box!" exclaimed Patty. "Me impatient, indeed! Just for that, Little Billee, I'll put the date six months later."

"Later than what? I didn't know you'd decided on the date for the festal occasion. You told me last night you hadn't."

"I'm living up to the reputation for fickleness Helen has just wished on me," Patty laughed. "But I'll give you some tea, Billee mine, if you'd like it. Oh, what a lot of people! You make the tea, Nan!"

Patty left the table to welcome her new guests. Elise Farrington and Daisy Dow were followed by Chick Channing and Philip Van Reypen.

After introductions and greetings all round, Helen looked about her with an air of great satisfaction.

"This is as I thought it would be," she said, contentedly; "I do love afternoon tea, and we never have it at home. And I love people dropping in to it."

"Into the tea?" asked Channing.

"Yes, in to the tea, of course. And such lovely people! I want to know you all at once, but I suppose I'd make better headway by taking you one at a time."

"Take me first," begged Chick, who was much attracted by the sprightly newcomer.

"No, me," laughed Philip. "You can get acquainted with me in two minutes,—I'm the easiest of us all."

"Then I'll leave you till the last," smiled Helen. "After all, I believe I'll talk to the girls first. I want them to like me——"

"Oh, don't you care about the boys liking you?" said Patty.

"They will, anyhow," Helen retorted, and she sat down by Daisy and Elise, ignoring all the others.

"Tea, please," said Philip, sauntering over to Patty, who had returned to the tea-table.

"One lump or two?" she asked, holding the sugar tongs.

"One and a smile," he replied.

Gravely, Patty dropped one lump in his cup, equally gravely, she gave him an idiotic smile, that was merely a momentary widening of her mouth.

"Very pretty," commented Phil; "don't see how you manage such a sweet smile! The tea is 'most *too* sweet, I think. Give me another bit of lemon."

"Here you are," said Patty, spearing the lemon with a little fork. "Now, Philip, listen to me. I want you to do all you can to make it pleasant for Bumble,—I mean, Helen, while she's here."

"Of course I will. I'm always nice to your friends, you know that."

"I do know it, but I want you to be *specially* nice."

"All right. Say, flowers tonight,—candy to-morrow,—opera invitation as soon as I can manage it,—a theatre party,——"

"There, there, now don't overdo it! No;

she doesn't eat candy, but you may send some flowers."

" Some to you too."

" No; not to me——"

" Then not to her."

" Oh, Phil, you said you'd be nice! "

" Well, I will; to both of you. But not to Bumble—I mean, Helen, alone."

" But you mustn't send flowers to me, now that I'm engaged. Come here a minute, please, Little Billee."

" Yours to command," said Farnsworth, approaching.

" Tell Philip he can't send me flowers."

" Philip, you can't send Patty flowers," Farnsworth said, obediently.

There was a smile on his face, but in his voice there rang a note of command that angered Van Reypen exceedingly.

" I can *send* them," he returned, defiantly, " she needn't accept them."

" Leave it that way, then," Bill said, carelessly, as if the matter were of no moment. " Patty, come out to the dining-room a minute, will you, dear? "

Jumping up, Patty left the room without a glance at Philip.

Farnsworth followed her, and they went into the dining-room.

They were alone there, and he took her gently in his arms.

"What is it, Patty?" he asked. "Van Reypen been kicking over the traces?"

"Yes; he seems to think he—he likes me yet."

"Of course he does. How can he help it? But, my darling, there's to be no petty jealousy between us and him. I trust you, dear, too well, to think for a minute that you'd listen to him if he says things that you don't want to hear. Now, never think it will bother me, for it won't. You love me, don't you, Patty?"

"Yes," she returned, and the blue eyes that met his left no room for doubt.

"Then, that's all right. Don't give him a thought. Darling, I've brought your ring."

With a smile of pleasure, Farnsworth produced a lovely ring. It was set with a single pearl, which he had told Patty suited her far better than a diamond.

"Do you like it?" he asked eagerly. "Oh, Patty Blossom, *do* you?"

"I think it the most beautiful ring I ever saw!" she replied, her eyes glistening, as he slipped it on her finger.

" My pearl," he whispered, close to her ear, " my Patty Pearl. This seals our betrothal, and makes you mine forever."

" Am I any more yours than I was before I had it? "

" No, you little goose! But this is the bond, —the sign manual——"

" Oh, Little Billee! *what* a joke! But I accept my bond,—I glory in it! Oh, Billee, what a beauty pearl it is! "

" The purest and best I could find,—for my own Patty Blossom. Now, I've bad news, darling."

" Bad news soon told, Br'er Fox," smiled Patty, quoting from her well-beloved Uncle Remus. " What is it? "

CHAPTER III

"IT'S this," said Farnsworth, looking serious. "I have to go to Washington."

"Good gracious!" exclaimed Patty, "one would think you were booked for Kamschatka or Siberia, the way you say it!"

"But I mean, I have to go there to stay."

"How long?"

"Indefinitely. I've no idea how long; also— I may have to go further yet."

"Over there?"

"Yes. But that's not likely at present. However, it's bad enough to go to Washington. How can I leave *you?*"

"I'll go, too."

"No, dear, that won't be practicable. I shall be in the University Camp, drilling engineers, I suppose, but I want to do more and bigger things than that. I can't tell you all about it, Posy Face, but as soon as I get further orders I'll know better where I'm at."

Captain Bill

" Are you bothered and troubled, my Billee Boy? "

" I am, Patty. I don't want to worry you with it, dearest, and you couldn't understand it all, anyway, but there is a lot of backbiting and undermining and wire-pulling in Washington, and it even mixes into Army and Navy matters."

" Then you'll have to be an undermining engineer, won't you? "

" Patty! You little rogue! You'd make a joke out of anything, I believe."

" 'Course I would! Now, Billee, you mustn't look so down-hearted. You've got me for a joy and a comfort,—not for a burden and a—a millstone about your neck! "

" I like to have you about my neck, all right, —but you're a featherweight, not a millstone."

" Where will you be? What's this camp? "

" The Engineering Corps, you mean? Oh, well, there are a lot of units,—Camouflage, Foresters, Gas and Flame, Wireless, Telephone,——"

" There, there, that'll do! I'm bewildered. Which are you to be in? "

" That's the trouble. It looks to me as if I'd be in the Searchlight gang——"

" What do you know about searchlights ! "

" Nothing.   To be sure I've invented one—"

" Oh, Billee, have you?   And you never told me ! "

" Hadn't time.   There's only time enough, when I'm with you, to tell you what I think of you."

" What do you think of me ? "

The lovely face was wistful and sweet, the blue eyes shone with affection and the scarlet mouth drew down a little at the corners, for Patty saw by Farnsworth's pained expression, that he was really disturbed at their coming separation and the uncertainties of his future.

" I think," the big man spoke, slowly, " I think you're the loveliest thing God ever made. A thousand times too good for a big brute of a man like me——"

" You don't treat me like a brute," observed Patty.

" No; I treat you as I think of you,—a lovely rose petal of a girl,—who ought not to hear of wars or rumours of wars——"

" Nothing of the sort, William Farnsworth ! If I were that, I'd deserve to be put under a glass bell, and left there to die of asphyxiation ! I'm *not* a silly roseleaf,—I'm a willing, working patriot! Why, I'm as energetic as—as Molly Pitcher or Barbara Frietchie—or Joan of Arc!"

"That's right, dear, that's the right spirit! But you know, Pattibelle, you're not physically fitted to go on the rampage, as your flashing eyes indicate. You're the sort who must ' stay, stay at home my heart and rest; homekeeping hearts are happiest.' "

"Little Billee, you do quote the beautifullest poetry! Where *do* you pick it all up?"

"Oh, I've a store of it somewhere in the top of my head. And I mean no disparagement of your enthusiasm, Patty, but you can't do hard work, and so——"

"And so I must knit and knit and knit, I s'pose! Billee, dear, when you go to Washington why can't I go too, and work in the Canteen Department?"

Farnsworth smiled at her. "Do you know what the Canteen Department is?"

"Not exactly; but Louise Dempster has gone to it,——"

"Oh, it's the Commissariat Department, but it's no place for you——"

"Why?"

"There, there, don't snap my head off! Only

because you're not robust enough for the work. If you're going in for real help, there's always the hospital or ambulance work."

"I—I couldn't, Billee!   I—I'd faint, I know! Oh, dear, I'm no good, and never was and never will be!"

"Not so very much good to your Uncle Samuel I admit," and Farnsworth grinned at her, "but a whole heap of good to one of his humble citizens."

"Which one?"

"This one!" and Bill grabbed her in his arms.

"Drop me," Patty murmured, half smothered in his shoulder, "somebody's coming!"

"Let 'em!"   But he set her down and began to speak seriously.   "You do all you can for the Red Cross, dear, and that will be your share.   Now, don't worry over it, or think you ought to get into the game in any other way. You can't do it, but you can and do accomplish a whole lot,—besides your knitting.   Blossom Girl, remember *I'm* in this world, as well as the rest of the U. S. A. and you'll give *me* of your love and fealty and——,"

"Do you think I will, Sweet William?"

Patty's very soul looked out of her earnest

[46]

eyes, and Farnsworth kissed her reverently, " I know you will, darling. Now, you've helped me a lot already by your cheery and pleasant attitude about my going away——"

" But I don't know all about it yet."

" I don't know much myself. I'll have further instructions soon——"

" And a uniform?"

" Of course. I'll rank as a Captain, and——"

" Oh, Captain Bill! How I will love you then! Come in the other room, I must tell of it! Nan, Billee's going to have a uniform!"

" Heavenly!" cried Helen Barlow. " Oh, I adore uniforms! And Mr. Farnsworth will be stunning in one!"

" You may call him Bill, if you like," said Patty, in the generosity of her enthusiasm.

" All right," said Helen, " but I don't think it suits him. William is much more dignified."

" Make it William, then," and Farnsworth smiled at the saucy-faced girl.

" Captain Farnsworth is the best," said Elise. " The title becomes you, Bill, and I know the uniform will."

" I'm going to have a uniform too," said Van Reypen, " won't it become me?"

[47]

"Me, too," chimed in Channing. "I'm expecting to be ordered to France any minute."

"Why, Chickering Channing! I didn't know that," cried Patty. "What are you?"

"I'm an *Officier de liaison.*"

"What in the world is that?"

"It's really nothing but an interpreter. But the French term is so much more impressive."

"Indeed it is. What do you interpret?"

"Words otherwise unintelligible."

"But I don't understand—"

"Then I'll be pleased to interpret for you. You see, if a French soldier wants to confide a state secret to an English-speaking comrade, and if he doesn't know a word of English, nor the other chap any French,—what's to be did?"

"Oh, I see!" cried Helen, "they call you in!"

"Exactly, Miss Barlow. And being conversant with and fluent in all known tongues,—I'm just a walking Tower of Babel."

"A walking dictionary, you mean," laughed Helen. "I think that's a pretty fine position you hold. I never heard of it before. What's your rank?"

"Lieutenant,—very much at your service,

Mademoiselle. Shortly, I shall don my khaki, and then I hope, at last, I'll be respected by my fellow men."

"That's so, Chick," said Patty, mercilessly, "you've always been such a cutup—well, of course, you were respected,—but nobody really stood in awe of you. But a Lieutenant,—oh, I'm proud of my friends!"

"Isn't it glorious!" cried Helen, and she flew to the piano and began playing patriotic airs. They all joined and a brave chorus of young voices rang out the avowal that the Yanks were coming over there!

So enthusiastically did Helen pound the keys that her hair shook loose from its pins and came tumbling round her shoulders.

"Now, now, Bumble," remonstrated Patty, "don't do so,—it isn't done! Here, I'll fix it for you."

But Helen only laughed, and nimbly twisted up her tousled locks, and thrust hairpins in to hold them in a hard and unbecoming knot at the back of her head.

"It doesn't look a bit nice," Elise warned her. "Better let Patty rearrange it."

"Nope, I don't care," and the wilful girl kept on playing and laughed as she shook her head.

The shaking sent her hair down again, and this time Patty determinedly went to her and dressed it for her.

"Sit still, you naughty!" she said, herself shaking with laughter. "Oh, Bumble, you haven't grown up a bit!"

Patty did up her cousin's hair prettily and skewered it firmly into place with many hairpins, and it didn't come down again.

"And are you going down to Washington, too, Chick?" Daisy Dow asked.

"Sooner or later, yes. That's the road to all war glory."

"And you don't know when?"

"You nor I nor nobody knows. You see, Daisy, in war affairs nobody knows anything and if they do they're not allowed to tell it."

"But just among us,—we wouldn't tell anybody."

"The walls have ears," said Chick, mock-dramatically.

"And Rumour has a thousand tongues," added Farnsworth, "it's a dangerous combination."

A week later the two went to Washington. Sent for nearly at the same time, Farnsworth and Channing were to go to Washington, though their work there was widely different.

The night before their departure, there was a gathering of the clan at Patty's home.

Farnsworth begged her not to have others there on their last evening together, but Patty's wise little head thought it better to have a party.

"You see," she said to Nan, "if I spend the evening alone with my Billee Boy, he'll be so sad and blue, and I'll be so weepy and red,— we'll have an awful time! It's a whole lot better to have the crowd here and let him go off in a blaze of glory! Patriotism is good for homesickness."

And, too, Patty was trying to entertain Helen pleasantly, and so she made many little parties for her.

The plan of entertaining the other soldiers was postponed until they could do no more for their own friends, and the little party to speed their parting, though small, was gay and festive.

"A dance," Patty decided. "I don't want just a sit-around, woeful, sighful time. A good, lively dance, and a nice supper, and then——"

Patty choked, and Nan seeing the springing tears, quickly began to discuss details of the supper.

The evening came, and Patty dressed in white, went to Helen's room to make sure she· was in proper order.

"Why, Helen Barlow!" she exclaimed; "if you're not an apple-pie pink of perfection! Not a bow coming off, and your hair positively looks as if it would stay put!"

"Don't tease me, Patty. Truly, I'm trying to do better,——"

"You dear old thing! I was a wretch to seem to tease you. Wait till this ball is over and you get off that very bewitching frock, and I'll give you a kiss of forgiveness!"

Helen looked very pretty in her evening dress of soft, thin pink, with touches of silver lace, and silver slippers.

"You're a fairy," said Patty. "How that frock becomes you. Now, be gay and festive, won't you, Helen, honey, for I feel as if I should burst into a flood of tears every minute!"

"Go on down, Patty," said Helen, drawing back, " I hear Billee's voice, and he'll want you alone."

"No; I can't. If I do, I'll cry. Come along."

So both girls ran down stairs, and shrieked with delight at the sight of Farnsworth in uniform.

"I knew you'd be stunning," said Helen, "but I didn't know you'd look like a Herculean statue!"

"He doesn't," cried Patty, "he looks like a—a General! He ought to be—oh, what do you call it when you have your statue taken?"

"Sculped," said Helen.

"Yes, that's it! He ought to be sculped in marble or bronze or whatever is most used for statues this year!"

"There, now, kiddies, run away and play," said Farnsworth, towering to his full height and looking every inch a soldier.

"No sir," declared Patty, "we want to look at you. Turn around."

Then Channing came, and he, too, was resplendent in his new khaki, and the girls praised his appearance.

"Drink it in, Bill," Chick said. "It'll be a long time before we get any more of this sort of thing! Somepin tells me the people we're

going amongst won't pay any special attention
to our uniforms."

" How can they help it? " cried Helen; " why,
I don't believe any of the United States Army
will look half as well as you two! You're—
you're superb! "

A bit embarrassed, Channing tried to turn
the subject, but Farnsworth laughed good-
humouredly.

" Let 'em rave, Channing. They enjoy it,
and I guess we can stand it——"

" Pooh," Patty said, " you're tickled to death
to be so admired! Here comes Elise, now
you'll get more flattery."

And then the other guests came and the party
soon was in full swing.

Patty was among the gayest there. Her eyes
shone and her smile was merry and sweet. But
a flush showed on each pink cheek, and Farnsworth kept watch of her as she danced or
engaged in light banter with the young
people.

Helen Barlow was frankly delighted with the
party. She was a belle, indeed, for she was a
charming dancer and her never-failing fund of
fun and laughter kept her partners enchanted.

" I like to dance with you," she said to Farnsworth, " 'cause you're so big. It's like dancing with one of the statues in the park."

" Why do you girls look on me as a statue? " he returned, laughing. " There's nothing statuesque about me."

" No; not that, it's your heroic size——"

" I hope that's not *all* my heroism! "

" I hope so, too: But are you going to need heroism? Bravery, I mean, and courage and all that. I thought you were only going to teach the young engineers how to shoot."

" That's part of my duty, but there may be other work cut out for me."

" That's what Patty thinks. She thinks,— because you can't tell her all about it,—that you're going to be called to some fearful danger——"

" Oh, come now, Helen, she doesn't think that, does she? "

" Yes she does. She didn't exactly tell me so, but she can't hide it from me. I can read that girl pretty well."

" So can I."

" Yes, but you don't see her off her guard."

" I know what you mean. Just now, she is trying her best to be gay; trying so hard, indeed, that she's overdoing it."

"Yes, that's what I mean. You can tell by the way she laughs. A little hysterical giggle, —that's not like Patty's own hearty chuckle!"

"You're right, Helen; and you're a good friend to Patty. I'm so glad you're here with her. Can you stay some time?"

"Yes, as long as she wants me."

"Then look out for her, won't you? She's a frail little thing, and her heart and her energies are too big for her physique."

"That's so, Bill. But I'll look after her,— all she'll let me. She has a strong will, I can tell you."

"You two are talking about me, I can sense it!" cried Patty herself, coming up to them.

"We are," said Bill, "and I'm going to talk to you, instead. Helen, I see your next partner coming hot haste to claim you, so I'm going to take Pattibelle aside and treat her to a small lecture."

Willingly Patty went with him, and he led her to the little room which was her father's den.

There chanced to be no one there, so Farnsworth closed the door after them, and then gently took her in his arms.

"Dearest," he said, "you must be careful of my own little Patty girl while I am away."

" But I don't want you to go," she whispered, her lip trembling.

"I know it, dear, and I don't want to leave you. But we're always going to obey the call of duty, aren't we, Patty mine?"

" Y-yes,——"

"Then listen, sweetheart. You mustn't exaggerate our parting. I'm only going to Washington——"

"I know—but—you may be sent to France——"

" Don't cross that bridge until you come to it. Now, my own,—my blessed little girl, I'm going now."

" Now?"

"Yes, if I stay here you'll go all to pieces pretty soon. So I'm going now, and I'm going to say good-bye, cheerfully, even calmly,—because it's better so. Then you go back to the party and be as gay as you like, and forget our case entirely. Trust me, dear little girl,—it's better so."

Patty realised the truth of Farnsworth's words. She was under great nervous strain, and after his departure, she knew she could regain her poise and better conceal and control her feelings.

" You're right, you dear old Billee. I'm a little fool, but I can't help it. I oughtn't to have planned this affair the way I did, but I didn't realise,——"

" Of course you didn't, and you overestimated your own power of will. Now, my love, my little sweetheart, kiss me once, for soldier's luck, and then I'll go,—and you must bid me good-bye with a smile,—a smile that I'll carry with me always."

Silently, solemnly, Patty raised her face to his, and bending down, Farnsworth kissed the sweet lips that quivered beneath his touch.

It almost unnerved him, but, determinedly, he smiled at her, and said, cheerily, " I'll write often and so must you, and,—why, my goodness, Patty,—I'll be back soon on leave, and we'll laugh at this tragic parting."

" No; we won't laugh at it my Little Billee, —no, not that,—but,—we'll try to smile."

" And succeed! Show me how, *now*."

Patty smiled with real cheer, and clasping her quickly, Farnsworth gave her one big, farewell kiss, and rushed out of the door, closing it behind him.

CHAPTER IV

THE BOYS IN KHAKI

"OH, it was the best plan, but I did hate to have him run off like that."

"Of course you did, Pattykins, but you would have flown into forty conniption fits if he had stayed longer. I saw you, and you were getting all nervous and 'stericky!'"

"I was not! You exaggerate so, Bumble, and I won't stand it! I was upset, of course, at the thought of his going, but I had absolute control of my nerves. It was all my own fault,—having the party, I mean."

"You had the party for me, my child. Don't think you can fool your grandmother! But it's all right, and I promised that Sweet William of yours that I'd chirk you up, and keep you so interested and amused that you'd forget his very existence,—let alone forgetting his absence. Besides, there's a strong belief current in the best circles that absence makes the heart grow fonder."

" It can't ours,—we're all the fond there is, now ! "

" Turtle-doves! Well, give me a bit more chocolate, and we'll call it square."

The two girls, in boudoir gowns and caps, were having their morning chocolate in Patty's room, and had eagerly been rehearsing and discussing the party of the night before.

Helen's pretty hair was tousled and her cap askew, as, perched cross-legged on a couch, she nibbled toast and sipped chocolate contentedly.

Patty, fresh and tidy as a rose, sat near by and did the honours of the breakfast tray.

" You see," she said, absent-mindedly piling sugar into Helen's cup, " I've decided to be sensible about this thing. I'm not going to——"

" You're going to get a Food Controller after you if you are so lavish with that sugar! For Heaven's sake, Patty, stop! That's the third spoonful! "

" Is it? I wasn't looking. As I say, I'm going to be sensible about Little Billee's going away. He's got to go, and so I may as well make up my mind to it."

" Sensible, indeed! Yet it doesn't seem to me such a marvellous triumph of intellect or such a phenomenal force of will that brings about that resolve!"

"In one more minute I shall throw a pillow at you, Bumble! I guess if you were engaged to the biggest man in the world, you wouldn't let him walk off to war——"

> "He's going with the whole
> Of his patriotic soul,
> At the call of his country's flag!"

sang Helen, trilling the refrain of a song they had all sung the night before.

"Yes, that's it. And what am *I* to stand out against Uncle Samuel?"

"That's right, be patriotic and you will be happy,—you are a nice child, Patty."

"*You* would be, if you weren't so silly!"

"Me silly! Ah, well, better judges are better pleased!"

Helen rolled her eyes skyward, in mock resignation, and then began to finger over Patty's engagement book.

"To-night, Elise's party," she read; "will that be fun?"

"Oh, yes, she has lovely parties. And, write it in there for me, Bumble, we've decided on

[61]

next Monday night for a party for the boys in khaki."

" All right, I'll put it down.   Who did the deciding? "

" Phil and I, last night.   He says he'll make application to the Y. M. C. A. committee or something and have them send us the pick of the lot."

" How funny!   The best-looking ones?   Do they have to pass an exam for it? "

" Don't be idiotic!   Let me tell you, the most desirable ones are merely the ones who most need a little pleasure or entertainment."

" How can they tell? "

" Oh, I don't know.   Perhaps the ones who are farthest from home and mother,—or, who have been ill,—— "

" Or parted from their best girls? "

" Yes, those are the saddest cases, of course! "

" Well, go ahead, I'll be best girl to 'em."

" You see, Philip knows the—the—— "

" Chaplain? "

" Well, the somebody, who will pick out the boys,—soldiers and sailors both, and I've agreed to entertain a few every Monday night, for the present, anyway."

" You're a good girl, Patty; you're all right! "

The Boys In Khaki

"Oh, *thank* you, dear, for your generous praise!"

"Yes; I foresee these parties will so interest and entertain you, that I'll not have to work so hard to keep my agreement with your big man to divert your saddened and aching heart."

"My heart's outside your jurisdiction,—and beside, I'm doing this party to entertain you. You know, one can't have a guest without making strenuous efforts to keep said guest merry and bright, please!"

"True, yes, true! But, give me half a chance, and I'll entertain myself. Give me a pleasant home to visit, a lovely hostess, like——"

"Oh, *thank* you!"

"Like Nan, and a few young men, and I'll ask nothing further."

"I seem to be left out of your scheme of things!"

"No, no! my angel child, not so, but far otherwise!"

The vivacious visitor flung aside her pillows and jumped up to embrace Patty in a whirlwind flash of affection. Greatly given to chaffing, Helen was truly fond of Patty, and the two were congenial and affectionate.

"Now, one more tiny pour of chocolate, and

one more popover, and my matutinal meal is finished," Helen said, resuming her seat.

"Oh, Bumble! You know you are welcome to all you want, and more too, but—but I thought you *did* want to—to———"

"To help this too, too solid flesh to melt? Well, so I do,—but Patsy, poppet, your talented cook does make such delectable dainties that I can't resist. Just a teenty-weenty drop of choclum, there's a dear, sweet cousin-girl!"

Patty laughed and gave Helen another cup full of the delicious cocoa, and turned her glance aside, as a popover was lavishly buttered.

The morning mail came then, and as Jane brought the girls their letters, Helen took hers, and suddenly gave a deep and hollow groan.

"What's the matter?" asked Patty, but half-heartedly, as her mail contained a letter from Little Billee, which she was eagerly devouring.

"Matter enough!" wailed Bumble, "that botheration, that pest of my existence, that everlasting nuisance, Chester Wilde, is coming here!"

"Here? When?"

"I dunno. Soon, he says. Today, most

likely. I think I'll telephone him not to come."

" Why? Why don't you let him? "

" Oh, he's such a persistent—er, wooer."

" Don't you care for him, Helen? "

" Not enough to marry him, as he insists I must do."

" Oh, well, let him come. I'll talk to him, if you don't want to. When may he be expected? "

" Today, I suppose. Oh, of course, he'll only come to call,—and I forbid you, Patty, to ask him to stay to dinner—or to come again."

" Wowly-wow-wow! What a cruel fair she is! All right, Bumble, dear, just as you say. And now, scoot back to your own room,— unless you want more chocolate? "

" N-no," and Bumble looked longingly at the tray. " No,—no! of course not! "

Patty laughed, and gently pushed her visitor out of the room, lest temptation again overcome her.

The Monday evenings planned for the enjoyment of the boys in uniform began to take shape and rapidly acquired considerable proportions.

Philip Van Reypen was a fine organiser and

Helen Barlow ably seconded his efforts, while Patty agreed and helped in matters of detail.

Elise was interested and there were half a dozen more of their own crowd ready to help in any way available. Chester Wilde had put in an appearance and Patty liked him from the first. A quick-witted, pleasant-mannered young man, himself engaged in some clerical war work, he declared his willingness to come over from his home in Philadelphia and help with the Monday night parties.

Helen Barlow's pretended dislike of him was merely coquetry, Patty surmised, and then as the elder Fairfields approved of young Wilde, he soon became a frequent and welcome visitor.

Patty adhered to her plan of giving the enlisted men evenings of real pleasure, and entertainment that was enjoyable to educated and cultured minds. For the first evening, they planned a series of Living Pictures, for, said the sagacious Patty, "give 'em something to look at that's pretty and they're bound to like it!"

Elise Farrington and Daisy Dow were enthusiastic workers, and Mona and Roger Farrington promised any help asked for.

The Boys In Khaki

As Farnsworth and Chick Channing were both gone away, the circle of Patty's friends was depleted as to men, but Chester Wilde was a good help and two or three other men were invited to assist.

Philip Van Reypen was still in the city, and his great efficiency and good taste and judgment made him a valuable ally for the cause.

He and Patty planned the pictures, for Helen Barlow knew nothing of such matters and Chester Wilde was better at carrying out orders than originating plans.

"What do you think of this scheme," Van Reypen asked of Patty as they began on the actual selection of subjects. "Say, three pictures,—tableaux, you know, and have each of them introduce a bit of entertainment of itself."

"Sounds fine," she agreed, "if only I had the least idea of what you're driving at."

"You will have. Here's the gist of it. Say, an Oriental scene. Ladies in rich Persian draperies and fallals posed about; men in the gorgeous Eastern robes affected by our heathen contemporaries; all the properties and effects in harmony,—you know I've oodles of that junk —and the whole scene glittering and radiant."

" Beautiful! Great! But is that all? "

" Not so but far otherwise. Now, after the eager audience have feasted their eyes on the sight, and you know, it isn't to be a motionless picture,——"

" Then it must be a motion picture! "

" It is, in this sense. The ladies and the men walk about, or languidly wave their peacock feather fans, or sink gracefully on divans, but of course, no words are spoken."

" Pantomime, then."

" Yes; rather like a pantomime. Well, then, in comes an Oriental juggler, who does tricks,——"

" I see! Oh, Phil, that's splendid! Just what I wanted! And he does real tricks,— good tricks,—and they interest the audience of themselves, and at the same time there's the beautiful scenic effect going on! "

" Yes,—a poor scheme,—but mine own."

" A fine scheme! Oh, I see enormous possibilities in it! "

" Then perhaps on another occasion, a Sylvan scene,—a woodland effect,—and in it give a bit of ' As You Like It,' or something of that sort. Another time, a Venetian scene, and you can sing with the gondoliers."

" Yes, yes, I see it all! "

" Oh, you do! Then you've no further need of my services."

" Don't be a silly! Of course I want you. I couldn't do any of it alone. How long before you go to Wilmington, or wherever you're going? "

" Dunno! but it won't matter. I can run up here often. An aviator's life is not a busy one."

" Really? Why isn't it? "

" Oh, it is, of course, in a sense. But there's not the same strenuous rush there is in other fields. You see we're not fly-by-nights, for one thing."

" Oh, yes, outside daylight hours you're free to play by yourself? "

" Perhaps not all of that, but, don't you worry, my lady, I'll play hookey, if need be, to get up here to look after your interests."

" All right. Now we can't put a whole lot of time and trouble on rehearsals and all that, you know."

" No; my idea was to have these things almost impromptu. Let us plan it all out pretty well beforehand, and then let the performers each time come early, and get posted as to their parts, and the star performer will do the rest."

"Star performer?"

"Yes; I mean, each time have an entertainer, like the juggler——"

"A professional?"

"Not necessarily. I know a chap who does wonderful legerdemain, who'd be glad to come to entertain Our Boys."

"Oh, yes, I see. And I'll sing."

"Yes, you can sing, as special character in some tableau, don't you see? You could be a mermaid or a Lorelei, sitting on a rock."

"With a lute?"

"Yes, and your hair down, and a gold comb and a mirror, while you comb your shining goldilocks."

"Nixy! Not my hair down. All the rest, but now I'm engaged, I've put away childish things."

"Pshaw, don't be a silly! But never mind those details. And, too, if you don't fancy the mermaid rôle, have a bit of a scene about ' tenting tonight on the old camp ground,' and you can come on as a Red Cross nurse, and sing——"

"Oh, yes, and the boys in khaki can help make up the picture!"

[70]

The Boys In Khaki

" 'Course they can. And another time, we'll get up a ship scene, I don't know just how yet, but I'll plan it——"

" We could have the mermaid come to the side of the ship."

" Ah, coming around to the mermaid rôle, are you? Well, those schemes are all right. Now, what shall we choose for the first one? "

" Not soldiers or sailors. Let them see some stunning show first."

" Oriental? "

" Yes, I guess so. Your idea of the juggler is splendid. He can come on the stage like those Hindoo fakirs, you know,——"

" Yes, that's what I meant."

" You know, there's not so very much room——"

" Want to go over to Elise's, and have it all in her casino? "

" N-no,—not at first, anyway. You see, Phil, I suppose it is nothing but pride and vain glory, —but *I* thought up this plan,—and I want to have it in my own home."

" So you shall! I don't blame you. If Elise wants to, let her get up something herself."

" Probably she will. But I want mine here."

" That's all right, Patty-girl. Why, there's

plenty of room. We needn't ask so very many guests,—say a dozen or so the first time, and see how it works out."

"Oh, we could accommodate twenty or twenty-four, I think. You see we'd use these connecting rooms, and this room would hold about thirty chairs."

"All right. Now, say we plan the scene. I've all that big chest full of Oriental costumes, you know, and we don't want very much in the way of actual scenery. A couple of divans heaped with pillows, and some of those hookah pipes standing round—then, the people in costume,—there's your setting,—see? Then, in comes your juggler, also in appropriate costume, and he does his tricks, and the people on the stage admire and applaud, and the people in the audience do likewise."

"Fine! And afterward, we have a little feast, and a little dance, and maybe sing a song or two for a good-night chorus."

"That's the ticket! Now, for the list of those who take part, and a few details of that sort, and our preliminary work is done!"

CHAPTER V

A FIRE-EATER

THE Monday night party was in full swing. A stage had been erected and the spectacle that was seen as the curtain rose was of " more than Oriental splendour."

Heavy draperies, potted palms, strange braziers and lanterns, pillowed divans,—all formed a brilliant and interesting picture of an Eastern interior.

Richly garbed ladies sat at ease while slaves waved peacock feather fans above their bejeweled heads. Stalwart men stood about, picturesque in their embroidered tunics and voluminous mantles.

The movement of the scene increased. Slaves entered with baskets of fruits, musicians came and made weird music, and dancing girls appeared and gave graceful exhibitions of their art.

Patty was one of these. In a charming costume of thin, fluttering silks and gauzy veils,

she went through the slow swaying steps of a
characteristic dance, and enthralled the appreciative audience.

She had indeed achieved her desire to give
her guests something different from the average
evening entertainment. The young men in
khaki and in blue, who sat watching, were
breathlessly attentive and applauded loudly and
often.

The whole assemblage was gay and merry.
The elder Fairfields were excellent hosts, and
chatted with the uniformed guests until even the
shy ones felt at ease. Roger and Mona Farrington, too, assisted in this work of getting
acquainted, and the result was a pleasant, chatty
atmosphere and not merely a silent audience.

"Good work!" said Roger, approvingly, to
a khakied youth, as Patty executed a difficult
pirouette.

"You bet!" was the earnest reply. "I've
seen some dancing, but never anything to beat
that! Is she on the regular stage?"

"Oh, no. She's the daughter of the house.
But she's a born dancer and has always loved
the art."

"Don't wonder! She puts it all over anybody I ever saw! And the whole colouring,—

the scene, you know,—well, it'll be something
to remember when I'm back in camp. A thing
like that stays in your mind, you know, and I'll
shut my eyes and see those furling pink veils as
plain, 'most, as I do now. What a beautiful
girl she is."

His tone was almost reverential, and Roger
instinctively liked the simple straightforward-
ness of his comment.

" Yes, and as lovely as she is beautiful. She's
engaged to a Captain, and it's hard luck that
he has to be away from her."

" It's all of that! Hullo, look who's here! "

Among the people on the stage there appeared
a strange figure. It was a man of swarthy
countenance, garbed in pure white draperies, so
full and flowing, that he resembled the pictures
of the prophets. He walked slowly to the
centre of the stage, and made deep salaams to
the characters there assembled, then turned
and bowed low to the audience. His snow-
white, coiled turban almost swept the floor as
he gracefully bent in greeting. Then he rose,
and began to chant a strange weird incantation.

An assistant brought a small tripod filled with
various paraphernalia, and the juggler began
his tricks.

Patty-Bride

They consisted of the most mystifying legerdemain and magical illusions, for the performer, as Philip had assured Patty, was an expert, though not a professional.

The soldier boys and sailor boys were delighted, and watched closely in their desire to see how the tricks were done.

And this paved the way to their still greater satisfaction, for the accommodating magician acceded to several urgent requests and explained his tricks.

To be sure, it detracted from the mystery, but it added to the interest.

One of his startling deeds was this.

An attendant brought to the magician a small iron dish filled with kerosene oil. With an eager smile, as of delighted anticipation, the juggler, who spoke no word, made motions for his aid to light the oil.

This was done, and the flames proved it to be real oil and really burning.

Then, taking an iron spoon, the magician dipped out a spoonful of the blazing oil and putting it in his mouth swallowed it with great apparent relish and enjoyment.

He nodded his head and smacked his lips in praise of this strange food, and made a gesture of wanting more. Obligingly, the attendant offered him the iron bowl again, and again a spoonful of blazing kerosene was gobbled up by the hungry feeder.

" My stars! " cried one of the audience, " I've heard of fire-eaters, but I never expected to see one! Have another dip, old chap! "

Smiling acquiescence, the juggler repeated his startling partaking of the oil, and seemed to like it quite as much as ever.

" Well, I'll give up! " cried the interested observer, who had spoken before. " Do tell us how you do that! I'd rather know that than eat a square meal myself! "

Dropping for the moment his rôle of pantomimist, the juggler said, " I will tell you, for it is an interesting trick. For years,—ages, even, the Hindus mystified and deceived people by pretending to be fire-eaters. The ignorant onlookers, of course, believed that the fakirs really ate fire,—hot coals, blazing oil, or burning tow.

" But as a matter of fact, it was all trickery, and deception of the simplest kind. You must know the ignorant people of the Far East are much more gullible and easily deceived than our own alert, up-to-date modern and civilised citizens. And, yet, even among ourselves, it is not easy to understand the fire-eating illusion. This is real kerosene, it is really lighted, you have seen my apparent relish of it. Now can any one explain how it is that I take spoonful after spoonful, yet my mouth is not burnt?"

Nobody could guess, and one after another said so. The young men were losing their shyness and self-consciousness in their interest.

"Spill it, boss," urged one, "give us the right dope!"

"Yes, I'd be glad to be informed as to the *modus operandi*," said another, who was of a different mental type. Indeed, it was all sorts and conditions of brains that were striving to see through this absorbing problem.

Patty, still in her place on the stage, looked keenly into the upturned faces.

"Dear, brave boys!" she thought to herself; "sooner or later, going 'over there' to fight for us and our cause! I am glad to give them a little cheer and fun as occasion offers."

The elder Fairfields felt the same way, and all who were helping Patty in her plan were conscious of a thrill of gratification at the success of it, so far.

"I've seen it on the vaudeville stage in Paris,"

one different looking youth spoke up. "It was slightly different in effect, but I suppose the same principle obtained."

"Doubtless," agreed the juggler, whose name was Mr. Peckham. "Now, I'll show you. The whole secret is that when I apparently take up a spoonful of oil, in reality, I only dip the spoon in and out again. It comes out blazing, to be sure, but really empty. It is merely the slight film of oil adhering to the spoon that blazes. However, this is quite enough to give the effect of a full spoon of kerosene on fire. Then, as I throw back my head, as if to swallow this flaming fluid, I really blow out the flame and I am careful not even to allow the hot spoon to touch my lips. But the audience, if the trick is quickly done, see what they expect to see. They are imbued with the idea that I am swallowing a spoonful of burning kerosene, and they therefore think I do so. It is over in a second,—I am swallowing, and smacking my lips, and it is taken for granted that I have done the impossible."

"Huh!" said the youth who had "wanted to know."

"Yes," returned Mr. Peckham, laughing, "it's 'Huh!' after the secret is told! No trick is as wonderful after it is explained as it is before."

" It is to me," said a more thoughtful man; " it's interesting to see how a mere optical illusion is believed to be real by thinking and attentive minds."

" Not only that," added Mr. Peckham, " but it's strange to realise how our eyes see, or we think they see, what we expect to see. You anticipated my fire-eating, you looked forward to seeing it, therefore, you thought you did see it."

" That's it, sir! After all, it's a sort of camouflage."

" Exactly! I give you something that looks like fire-eating, and you think it *is* fire-eating! Exactly."

Then he performed many other tricks; tricks with cards or with other paraphernalia; tricks with balls, swords, hats, all the usual branches of " magic " and the enthralled audience were so entertained and spellbound, that the time slipped by unheeded.

" Good gracious! " cried Patty suddenly, from her place on the stage, " isn't it getting late? "

" It's half-past eleven," Roger informed her, from the audience.

A Fire-Eater

" Then we must stop this magicking! I'm sorry, for I could watch it all night, but there's more programme yet!"

" Cut it out!" cried a youthful chap in sailor blue; " give us more hocus-pocus!"

" Not tonight," laughed Patty, and leaving her place, the whole tableau began to break up and the gorgeously attired Orientals came down among the audience and mingled as one group.

" I can't thank you enough," Patty said, pausing to speak to Mr. Peckham; " it's so kind of you, and I've been so interested!"

" Oh, it's nothing," asserted the kind and genial man, " glad to do it for Van Reypen's sake, for Our Boys' sake, and, most of all, Miss Fairfield, for your sake!"

Patty rewarded him with her best smile and ran away to look after the rest of her entertainment.

There was to have been music and some other matters, but it was now so late that it was time for the supper.

This was a simple but very satisfying repast and the men in uniform showed their appreciation of Patty's thoughtful kindness in this, as well as in the mental entertainment.

" I say, Miss Fairfield," a stalwart young man observed, " if you knew what all this means to us poor chaps, when we're miles removed from chicken salad and ice cream, you'd feel gratified, I'm sure."

" I do, Mr. Herron; I am truly glad I can please you but more grateful to you for your appreciation than you can possibly be for my invitation."

" Well, that's going some! " and the man laughed. " You see, Miss Fairfield, it's like a glimpse of another world to a lot of us. It is to me. Why, I come from out West, and I've never been in a home like this of yours. Oh, I don't mean to say we don't have 'em out West,—lots of our plutes roll in gold and all that. But *I* didn't. I'm of the every-day people, and my folks are good and honest, but plain. Not that I'm ashamed of 'em,—Lord, no! But I own up I'm pleased as Punch at this chance to be a guest in a fine house for once! "

" I hope not only for once, Mr. Herron," said Patty, who liked the frank young fellow. " I'd like to have you come again."

" You oughtn't to invite me,—you ought to take a different lot every time,—but, by jingo,

if you *do* ask me, I'm coming! You just bet
I am!"

Patty laughed and passed on talking gaily to
this one and that, asking questions about things
they were interested in and conversant with,
and in all, being a charming and sympathetic
little hostess.

Entertaining was Patty's forte, and she loved
it. Moreover, she could adapt herself with
equal ease to the most aristocratic and high-
bred society or to the plainer and more com-
monplace people.

As for these boys, she loved them, partly because of her patriot spirit, partly from her love
of humanity, and largely because now that her
own Billee was in the war, all war people were
dear to her.

After supper there was still time for a dance
or two, and the guests entered into this diver-
sion with zest. Naturally, Patty had many
would-be partners, and she divided her dances
in an effort to please many.

Helen, too, was a general favourite. The
young men liked the jolly girl and pretty Bumble laughed and joked with them, promising to
write letters to them and knit comforts for
them and to do numberless possible and im-

possible things when they were back in their camps, or wherever their duty led them.

Chester Wilde was present. He was an urgent suitor of Helen's, but tonight he tried with all his energies to help Patty in the plan she had undertaken.

At last, when most of the uniformed guests had departed, Wilde noticing the tired expression in Patty's eyes, led her to a cosy sofa and advised her to rest a little.

"I'll bring you some hot bouillon," he said, "and it will do you good. Let the rest of the girls speed the few parting guests, and you sit here and talk to me."

Patty agreed and soon they were affably chatting. As often, their talk was of Helen.

"Doesn't she look pretty tonight?" young Wilde asked, his eyes straying to the laughing face across the room.

"Yes, indeed, she always does," agreed Patty. "She's a darling thing, too, Mr. Wilde, and you mustn't be down-hearted because she flouts you sometimes. I know my little old Bumble pretty well and she's a great little scamp for teasing the people she likes best."

"It would have been all right, I'm sure," said the young man, moodily, "if she had stayed in

[84]

Philadelphia. But here, there are so many men about,—oh, I don't mean the uniformed men,—but a lot of others who are here at your house now and then, that I can't help feeling Helen will forget me."

"Nonsense! I won't let her. You trust your Aunt Patty! Why my middle name is Tact!"

"I know it, Miss Fairfield, I know all that, and you're awfully good to me, but,—oh, well, I s'pose I'm jealous."

"I s'pose you are," Patty laughed at him. "You wouldn't be any good if you weren't! But you know, faint heart and all that. Don't be faint-hearted, that's not the thing for a soldier, at all!"

"All right, I'll cheer up. You're a good friend, Miss Fairfield——"

"Oh, call me Patty, I'd rather you would."

"All right and thank you. First names for us, after this. Now don't think me silly, but, —won't you do all you can to—to——"

"To turn our Helen's heart in your direction? Indeed I will, Chester, and gladly. But, take my word for it, she likes you better than anybody else, right now."

"Oh, Patty, do you think so?"

"I know so. Bumble,—Helen, I mean, is a

[85]

dear, but she isn't quite sure of her own mind. Oh, don't you worry, Chester, my friend, all will yet be well."

"But look at her now. She's terribly taken with that chap named Herron. See her look at him!"

"The green-eyed monster has you in his grip, for sure! Come on, let's go and see what they're talking about."

Patty rose and Chester followed her to where Helen and Philip Van Reypen were eagerly talking to Mr. Herron.

"Yes," Herron was saying, "to train a thousand aviators usually means the smashing of more than a thousand machines. Why, every learner breaks up one or two airplanes before he's a flyer."

"Really!" said Helen, her eyes big with interest. "And how much do these airplanes cost?"

"Oh, about seven thousand dollars apiece."

"They do! What a fearful expense for the government!"

"The government does have fearful expenses, Miss Barlow,—or so I've heard."

"But that's something awful, old man," put in Van Reypen. "I'm going to be a flyer, and

I'll begin training soon. That's why I'm so keen on questioning you. Do I go up in the air at once?"

"No, sir. You begin on a machine that stays on *terra firma*."

"Then it isn't a flying machine at all," observed Patty, as she and Chester joined the others.

"Well, it is, except that it doesn't fly! But one learns all the motions on it, and the controls and the handling of winds,—and, oh, quite a few things about it. Then later on, one goes up——"

"What a sensation it must be!" cried Patty; "I'm just crazy to try it. May I go up with you, Phil, as soon as you've learned?"

"Not until I *have* learned. You'll take no chances with a novice, I can tell you."

"But I don't see," said Helen, "how a machine on the ground is anything like one in the air."

"It's difficult to explain," returned Herron. "But, you see, jets of air are blown through tubes, that simulate the currents of real air that affect the man higher up."

"Too many for me!" declared Helen, "my little two-cent brain refuses to grasp it!"

"We'll go down to see Philip perform as soon as he knows enough to show off," declared Patty. "Won't that be fun, Helen?"

"Yes; may we, Philip?"

"After I'm ready to show off, yes."

"Oh, you vainy!" cried Helen. "Never mind, we don't want to see you when you're just flying on the floor!"

"I really must fly from here," laughed Mr. Herron. "Such a gorgeous time, Miss Fairfield. May I come again?"

"Oh, I wish you would! Don't wait for a special invitation,—come at any time."

"He will," Van Reypen said, "I'll bring him. He and I will be associated, I find, in the Aviation Training Camp, and we'll often run up together,—mayn't we, Patty?"

"Yes, indeed; as often as you can manage to!"

CHAPTER VI

A SLEIGHRIDE

"READY, Bumble?" asked Patty, looking in at her cousin's room.

"Yes, in a minute."

"Oh, I know your minutes! They're half an hour long each! Here,—let me help you."

Patty straightened Helen's collar, fastened two hooks, found her gloves, tied her veil, and performed a few more odd services for her, and then held her fur coat for her to slip into.

"It looks like more snow, but Phil telephoned that we'd go anyway," Patty said: "Mona and Roger will meet us up there, and Mr. Herron will be there too."

"Perfectly fine! I love a sleighride, though goodness knows we get few enough of them nowadays."

"You won't love it, if we get snowed under, or snowbound at the Club."

"I shan't mind. We'll have Mona and

Roger for chaperons and we can stay till the storm is over. Philip says the house is lovely."

"Yes, the Timothy Grass Golf Club is a splendid place, and the winter casino,—The Playbox, they call it,—is most attractive. Oh, we'll have a good time whatever happens."

By way of entertaining Helen, Van Reypen had proposed a day at the Country Club, and his invitation was eagerly accepted. There was snow enough on the ground to make good sleighing, and the air was crisp, cold and clear. Warmly garbed for their trip, the two girls ran downstairs to find Philip awaiting them.

"Hooray for two plucky ones!" he cried; "I thought maybe you'd back out on account of the storm."

"Where's the storm?" asked Helen. "I don't see any."

"You wear rose-coloured glasses. There's snow in the air, some flying, and more waiting above, ready to come down. But not enough to hurt two such well-befurred Esquimoses! Come along, then."

The novelty of a real old-fashioned sleigh-ride was a great pleasure and as the fast horses flew along, the girls exclaimed at the new delight of such transportation.

A Sleighride

"Are Roger and Mona going in a sleigh, too?" asked Patty.

"Yes, I think so. They'll come later, as Mona just had a telegram that her father is coming to see her today."

"But she'll come to us, won't she?" Patty asked, quickly. "She's our chaperon, you know. It wouldn't do at all for Helen and me to go to the Club without her."

"Oh, yes, she said she'd come, as soon as her father arrives and she gets him comfortably welcomed. She's very fond of him, you know."

"Yes, and he's an awfully nice man. What time will we get back, Phil?"

"'Long about five o'clock or so. We won't reach the Club before noon. Then we'll have time for a game of indoor tennis or whatever you like, of that sort. Then luncheon, and in the afternoon there's time for a game of Bridge if you choose."

"Probably we won't do anything but sit around and chatter," opined Helen, who was not fond of games. "Mr. Herron is coming, isn't he?"

"Yes, my lady. But you mustn't flirt with him, or you'll turn his head completely."

"She has done that already," laughed

Patty; " Mr. Herron just sits and gazes at my fair cousin, whenever occasion offers."

" Nor can any one blame him for that. Look at the ice jam in the river! What a winter we're having, to be sure."

" A lovely winter, I think," Helen said, " I adore cold weather, and I don't mind snow. I like to feel it on my face."

" All the same," Patty put in, " I could do with less of it just now."

The white feathers were flying briskly through the air, and Patty cuddled her face deep into her high fur collar. She was not quite so fond of the elements as Helen, and felt the cold more.

> " The snow is falling all around,
>   It's falling here and there;
>   It's falling through the atmosphere
>   And also through the air."

Helen chanted the lines to an accompaniment of dashing the flakes from her veiled face.

> " The snow is falling all around,
>   And wonder fills my cup,
>   Whether, when it is all snowed down
>   We won't be all snowed up ! "

A Sleighride

Patty sang her parody, in a high, clear voice, and then returned to her depths of collar.

Then Philip took up the game:

" The snow is falling all around,
But you girls needn't fret;
We'll soon arrive where we are bound,
And you'll get warm,—you bet! "

"Lovely, Phil!" murmured Patty, "you do sing like a cherub!"

"Oh, well, I suppose my coloratura is a little off, but every time I open my mouth the snow snows in!"

"Ought to make liquid notes," said Patty.

"Oh, come now! If you're going to talk like that!"

"I can only sing of Greenland's Icy Mountains," Helen declared, and just then they came in sight of the Club house.

A huge structure it was, in a large park, and surrounded by trees and gardens. In summer it was a beautiful spot, but in winter some thought it even more so. The Golf Links showed great stretches of white and the bare black limbs of the tall trees made a picturesque foreground. The house itself, with glassed-in

[93]

veranda and storm doors, looked like a haven of refuge.

The girls ran inside, and were greeted by the sound of crackling flames in a great fireplace.

"I do think a Club is the nicest place!" exclaimed Helen, as she sat down on a fireside settle. "And this one has such a cheery, hospitable atmosphere."

"Yes," agreed Patty, "but I don't see many people around. Aren't there very few, Phil?"

"Rather so. But it's an uncertain quantity, you know. Some days the place is crowded, and again nearly empty. It's always so in a Club."

"Where's Mona?"

"She'll come soon. I told you she'd be late. Don't fuss, Patty."

"No; I won't," and Patty smiled at him.

But she was anxious, for Patty was conservative by nature, and a close observer of the conventions. She was unacquainted at this Club, and if Mona shouldn't come, she felt a grave uncertainty as to what she could do. She and Helen couldn't stay the day there without Mona, and the storm was gaining in force.

"I wish you'd telephone," she said to Van Reypen, "and see if they've started."

A Sleighride

"All right, my liege lady, I will. Just wait a minute, till I get this numbness from my digits."

"Do let him get warm, Patty," Helen remonstrated; "the poor man is almost frozen, and you send him to telephone about nothing!"

"'Deed it isn't nothing! If for any reason Mona doesn't come, we must go right home, Helen."

"But don't cross the bridge before you come to it. At least, let me have a look around. I want to see that sun-parlour and that other palmy nook, over there! Oh, I think this the most fascinating place I ever saw!"

"It *is* charming. And I'm glad to be here, but I want things right."

"Patty, you're not unlike Friend Hamlet. You're always setting the world right."

"I know, Phil, but you don't stop to think. You know we two girls can't stay here without Mona or some married woman as a chaperon. It doesn't matter what you think; that's society's law and must be obeyed."

Patty's pink cheeks took on an added flush and her blue eyes grew violet, as they did when she was very much in earnest.

"I know, Patty; I know, dear. Why, I'm as

[95]

well acquainted with the conventions as you are. Do you suppose I want you to do anything not absolutely correct? But the Farringtons will come directly. They started later than we did, and the increasing depth of snow may make them longer on the road. But they're sure to come."

Phil's air of conviction reassured Patty, and she turned to the great blazing fire again, with a sigh of contentment. There were two or three Club members about, but save for those and the liveried footmen here and there, the place was deserted.

Helen, thoroughly warm, jumped from her seat and went about looking at the various attractive rooms.

"A wonderful library!" she said, returning from her tour of investigation; "I could be happy there all day, just looking at the picture papers and books."

"So could I," said Patty, "if we had somebody with us. Why didn't we bring Nan? That would have made everything all right!"

"Mona's sure to come soon," comforted Helen. "Let up, Patty, you make me tired with your fussing."

A Sleighride

Good-naturedly, Patty " let up " and said no more for the moment.

" Hello, people! " called a cheery voice, and a big figure in uniform came swinging in.

" Mr. Herron! " cried Helen, running forward to greet him. " I'm so glad you came! Did you come in your airship? "

" I wish I could have done so, for the going on the ground is something awful. This is sure one fierce storm! "

Patty went over and lifted a curtain to look out of the window.

" Oh-ee! " she cried out, " it's coming down thicker'n ever! How can Mona get here? They'll be snowbound, half way here! Phil, please go and telephone; I *must* know if they've started."

" Better go quick," laughed Herron, " before the telephone wires are down. It's that wet, heavy snow that weighs the wires down fearfully."

" All right," and Phil started for the telephone booth.

" They'll get here," opined Bumble; " you worry over nothing, Patty Pink."

" They can't get here unless they started some

time ago," Herron said; " the roads are getting worse every minute."

" Roger will manage somehow," Helen went on. " I know him of old,—and he isn't to be baulked by a few flakes of snow."

But Phil returned looking serious.

" They're not coming," he announced, briefly, meeting Patty's startled eyes squarely, but apologetically. " Not on account of the storm, but because Mona's father arrived, and he isn't well and Mona won't leave him. She says to tell you she's awfully sorry, but it seems her father is really pretty ill, and she can't get away."

" Then we must go right home," said Patty, very decidedly. " You know yourself, Phil, we two girls can't stay here without Mona—or somebody."

" Of course, I know it, Patty. Give me a minute to think. I hate to go home and give up our nice day here. Maybe we can fix it. I'll go and see the housekeeper."

" Oh, that would be all right, Phil," and Patty's lovely face broke into a smile. " If she's a nice motherly or auntly old lady, she'd do admirably! Go and see about it, do!"

A Sleighride

"Let me go," said Herron, "maybe I can fix it up."

He was gone a long time, but he came back smiling.

"The housekeeper isn't here," he announced, "she's gone off for a few days' holiday. Her present substitute is her daughter, a girl younger than you girls are. Also there's nobody who can play chaperon to a pair of lone, lorn damsels but one elderly specimen, who is by way of being a pastry-cook or something like that. However,——"

"Oh, all right!" cried Helen; "I don't care if she's a pastry-cook or a laundress if she only satisfies Patty's insane desire for a chaperon! Will she come? Will she stay by us till we go home?"

"She'll come to luncheon with us," said Herron, "and after that I think we'd better start for home. The snow is getting deeper, and though it looks as if the sun might break through the clouds any minute,—yet it may not, and the drifts are high, and——"

"You're a calamity howler!" cried Helen. "We're here, and we're safe and warm, and the pie lady will do quite well for a chaperon, and anybody who grumbles now, is a wet blanket and a pessimist and a catamaran! So, there, now!"

"All right," Patty laughed; "let me see the elderly dame, and if she passes muster, I'll stop growling like a bear and be so nice and amiable you won't know me!"

"I don't know you when you're anything but amiable!" declared Philip; "where's your friend, Herron? Trot her in."

"She's dressing," Herron returned. "She said she must doll up to meet the young ladies——"

"Did she use that expression?" asked Patty, severely.

"Oh, no! That's mine. She said she'd put on her other gown,—or something like that."

"I can't decide till I see her," Patty said; "if she's really all right, we'll stay. If not, you must take us right home, Phil."

"Your word is my law. When Patty says go, we all goeth! Whew! how it snows!"

"Never mind the snow," urged Herron; "no matter what the weather when we four get together! Now, what can we do in the way of high jinks? Anybody want to try the swimming pool?"

A Sleighride

"No, thank you!" and Bumble shivered at the thought. "Can we dance anywhere?"

"Not till after lunch," said Patty. "Dancing in the morning has gone out. Besides, it's nearly lunch time now. Let's knit for a while, —and not go jumping about."

"You're a dormouse, Patty. You'd rather nod over your knitting needles——"

"I don't nod over them! I knit faster than you do! Come on, start at the beginning of your needle, and I'll race you for five rows."

The girls settled themselves comfortably by the big fire, and opened their knitting bags.

"Now, I call this fine!" declared Herron; "what's nicer than to have you girls sit and knit and we men sit and look at you!"

"There's nothing nicer to look at," said Helen complacently, "on that we're all agreed. Now, make yourselves entertaining, and we'll call it square."

Pretty Helen's gay face bent over her khaki-coloured wool, and her needles clicked bravely in an effort to knit faster than Patty. And she did, but it was only a spurt. She dropped a stitch, and exclaimed, "Hold on, Patty, no fair your knitting when I'm picking up this stitch! You wait now!"

"Not so; a dropped stitch in time loses nine! Come on, hare, catch up with this old tortoise!"

Calmly, Patty proceeded with her steadily-moving needles, and again Helen made an hysterical burst of speed and caught up as to distance. But her wool snarled somehow, and Herron, trying to help her, made it worse, and the four hands that tried to untangle it only drew it into tighter knots.

Helen burst out laughing, and awarded Patty the palm.

"It's always so," she acknowledged. "I fly at a thing and tumble all over myself, and accomplish just about nothing. Patty goes about it leisurely, and comes in at the last, easily winner, and with a big lot of work to her credit."

"You flatter me, angel child," Patty smiled. "I knit because I love to knit, and I get a lot done, because I don't try to beat everybody else. There, how's that for a helmet? I rather guess some one of Our Boys will be glad to wear it!"

"I shouldn't mind myself," suggested Herron, timidly, and Patty replied at once, "Then you shall have it! I'll fit it to your head now."

A Sleighride

"You want mine, Philip?" asked Helen, as she industriously "picked back" a few stitches.

"Yes, if I may be allowed to wear out two or three others while yours is in process of construction."

"Wot rudeness! To think I should live to hear such! Well, just for that I'll put all the knots inside!"

"They'll make me think of you!"

"And I'll put a note in it,—that's often done."

"A note of thanks. If the girls did that, it would save many a poor soldier a lot of trouble! He could just sign it and send it off."

"How unsentimental and ungrateful you are! Why, the boys just love to get notes in their socks and sweaters and then they love to answer them. It's no hardship, I can tell you! I've had the notes!"

"You can't have had very many,—you're too young."

Helen gave him a laughing scowl at this fresh fling at her slow progress and then she threw down her knitting.

"Can't do any more, now. I've come to the place to cast on, and I forget how many, and I left my paper of directions at home, and——"

"All right, come with me, and let's go and hurry up our chaperon lady," said Herron, rising.

"Yes, do," urged Patty, who was in nervous anxiety about that matter.

"Patty's in a pucker!" sang Helen, "like little
    Tommy Tucker!
    What shall she eat? War bread and
    butter!
How shall she eat it, without a chaperon?
    Put her in a padded cell and let her eat
    alone!"

Helen's foolishness never annoyed Patty, and so she bade the two ambassadors proceed with their errand and Helen and Mr. Herron went off.

"Trust me, Patty," said Philip, after the others had left the room, "it will be all right. The snow is lighter now; and we'll go home directly after luncheon. I don't want you to be disturbed, and I do understand,—you know I do!"

"Yes, I know it," Patty replied.

CHAPTER VII

A QUEER CHAPERON

WHEN Mrs. Doremus was introduced, Patty's thoughts ran somewhat like this:

"Nice old lady; apple-cheeked, white-haired and quiet-mannered. A little shy, but well-bred and kindly. Old-fashioned dress,—or, rather it looks so, because it's so long. Why, it almost touches the floor. But, she's all right, and her big, tortoise-rimmed glasses give her quite an air of distinction."

Helen, on the other hand, paid little attention to the chaperon, save to greet her pleasantly and thank her for her presence.

The five went to the Club dining-room for luncheon. There were a few others at various tables, but no one with whom the girls were acquainted.

"I'm fairly brimming with happiness," Helen announced; "I've always longed to be at a big country club in winter, and I've never achieved it before."

"It's winter, all right," said Herron, looking out at the steady snowfall. "But the palms and flowers make this seem like an oasis of summer, screened in."

"Awful pretty room," and Helen looked round contentedly, as she finished her grape fruit. "And of a just-right temperature. I'd like to stay here a week."

"You *may* get your wish," and Mrs. Doremus smiled at her, "if this snow keeps on, I don't see how you *can* go back to the city today."

"Oh, my goodness!" cried Patty, "don't say such a thing! Remember, Phil, when we were snowbound at that queer old house in the country?"

"Do I remember! Why, we had the time of our sweet young life up there! I never ate such chicken pie!"

"Nor I. And those two quaint old ladies were a whole show themselves."

"Oh, this storm isn't going to be so very bad," Herron said; "I think it's lessening now. We'll go down this afternoon, all right, all right. I think, Miss Fairfield, you're anxious to get a letter from somebody!"

A Queer Chaperon

Patty blushed prettily. "Well, perhaps I am. I came away before mailtime, you know."

"But you had one yesterday," Helen told, "a big, fat one! That ought to last you for a while!"

"But that was yesterday! I want today's bulletin."

"Aha! A letter every day?"

"Yes, Mr. Herron, that's the way engaged people keep alive, when separated by this cruel war!"

"Never mind letters now," begged Van Reypen, "let's forget everybody who isn't here."

"And are you engaged to a soldier, my child?" Mrs. Doremus asked of Patty. The old lady had a low, gentle voice, and though she said little, she had a delightful manner and a smile that betokened a keen sense of humour.

"Yes, to Captain Farnsworth; but he isn't exactly a soldier. I mean, he doesn't expect to fight. He is an expert mining engineer, and his country seems to find a lot of work for him, without sending him to the front."

"Bill Farnsworth, the Westerner!"

"Yes; do you know him?"

"No; not at all. But I saw something about him in the paper,——"

"You did! Oh, what was it? I'm interested, of course, in anything pertaining to him or his work."

"I can't seem to remember; I can't exactly place it; but I recollect seeing his name. And are you, too, engaged to an enlisted man, Miss Barlow?"

"No," said Helen, "but I hope to be."

"Quite right! Next to serving one's country, is being the helpmeet of one who does. Have you,—ah,—selected——"

"No, my selective draft hasn't yet been made," and Bumble's jolly little face smiled broadly; "you see, there are so many fascinating men in the service,—indeed, 'most any man is fascinating in uniform."

"I wear uniform," said Herron.

"I know, but lots of others do, too, and every time I meet a new one I lose my heart to him."

"I fear me you're a sad coquette, Miss Barlow," and the chaperon beamed on her.

"I am a coquette," Helen admitted, calmly, "but not at all a sad one! Indeed, I'm as merry as a grig. Why, I get letters from lots of the boys in camp. Miss Fairfield is content with only one correspondent, while I have a dozen! I just adore to get their letters, and to send them things, and to write to them. The war is terrible, but it does give one *some* new and pleasant experiences. And I don't feel it my duty to lament all the time. My mission is cheering people up and cheering soldiers on."

"I make no doubt you're a grand success at it, too. And some day you'll decide to send all your letters to the same address, as Miss Fairfield does. Where is Mr. Farnsworth now, may I ask?"

"In Washington," Patty replied.

"And is he coming to New York soon?"

"I don't know, I'm sure." Patty spoke a little coldly, for Bill had cautioned her over and over again, never on any account to tell any one of his plans or to repeat anything he might write, which concerned military matters or might give war information of any sort.

"How you must long to know! I don't mean definitely, of course, but can't you hope to see him soon?"

An insistent tone in Mrs. Doremus' voice caused Patty to look up quickly, and she saw the keen eyes regarding her intently through the big glasses.

But though the old lady's interest might have

been a bit strong for such short acquaintance, Patty was too polite to resent that, and she laughed and said, " It's impossible to tell, with a soldier boy. One can only hope,—one may not expect."

" That's a philosophical attitude, my dear, and does you credit. Is Captain Farnsworth in the Engineers' Camp?"

" Yes," said Patty, this time with decided shortness; " how very nice this sweetbread is! I've always been so fond of them. But one oughtn't to serve them on a sweetless day, ought one?"

" Oh, Patty, what a silly joke!" chided Helen. " You mean a meatless day!"

" Both ought to be barred," smiled Patty; " also they ought not to be served on a breadless day!"

" It looks as if they wouldn't be served at all any more," said Herron; " let's gather these sweetbreads while we may!"

" And perhaps the war will soon be over, and then we can eat what we like," Helen suggested. " It will be over soon, you know, because of the eagles."

" What do you mean?"

" Yes, it's a true omen. You know down at

A Queer Chaperon

Beverly, New Jersey, long ago,—oh, during the Revolution,——"

" Is this a real honest-to-goodness, once-upon-a-time story?" asked Van Reypen.

" Yes, it is."

" Then I move we move to the sun-parlour, and have our coffee there. We'll take our coffee,—sugarless, if Patty says so,—and then we can hear the story, and then we must see about going home."

" Fine," Patty agreed. " Will you join us in this desperate scheme, Mrs. Doremus?"

" Don't think you must, if you're busy," interposed Herron. " I'm sure the ladies will excuse you if you have duties to attend to."

" I haven't," returned the chaperon, calmly. " I'll be glad to have the coffee and the story, if I am permitted."

" Surely," said Helen, jumping up, " come along, Mrs. Doremus; you and I will pick out the sunniest spot. Philip, bring Patty; and Mr. Herron, will you order the coffee served there?"

Helen slipped her arm through that of the grey-haired lady, and they walked away together.

Philip detained Patty as she was about to follow.

"Queer old party," he said, very low.

"Who? Mrs. Doremus? I rather like her."

"Well, I don't! Be careful what you say before her, and we must get away as soon as we can."

"Why, Phil, what do you mean?"

"Nothing particular. Only, don't let Helen persuade you to stay all the afternoon. It's nearly three now, and we must get away by four, at latest."

"All right, Phil, but I never knew you to look so scared. Why?"

"Don't fuss, Patty; go ahead and join the crowd; but remember not to answer personal questions."

Patty wondered what had come over Philip's mind, but she thought no more about it, rather glad than otherwise, that he was determined to go home so early.

They crossed the big foyer, and across a chair there, was a fur stole of Patty's which she had left there in case of need while in the house. She picked it up, exclaiming: "Why, here's my fur! I might have forgotten it!"

A Queer Chaperon

"Lend it to me, won't you, if you're not wearing it?" asked Mrs. Doremus. "I feel a bit chilly,—but, perhaps you do too?"

"Oh, no; I'm warm as toast. Use it, by all means. Let me put it round you."

Patty draped the long stole round the shivering shoulders, and Mrs. Doremus said, apologetically, "I'm not really cold, but I take precaution for fear of rheumatism."

"Certainly," Patty acquiesced, and then the coffee tray was brought and Patty did the honours.

"Sugar?" she asked of the chaperon.

"One, please; and may I be excused for a few moments? I've just thought of an order I meant to give, and the gaiety of our little party made me forget it. I don't mind if my coffee gets a little cool,—I like it better so."

Mrs. Doremus went off toward the housekeeping quarters, and the others made merry over their coffee cups.

"I don't see why you want to start right off, Philip," Helen demurred. "I think it's going to stop snowing just about now."

"Do you, my child?" said Van Reypen, serenely; "be that as it may, we stand not on the order of our going, but go at once,—instanter,—immejit,—all-in-a-hurry,—so soon as your coffee is despatched."

"But why?" and Helen pouted.

"Yours not to put that direct question. Yours not to make remarks. Yours but to get into your befurments and hie away to town."

"I'm not at all sure we can make it," said Herron, pouring himself another cup of the rich brown beverage.

"Oh, yes, you can," and the cheery voice of Mrs. Doremus sounded in the doorway. "This my cup? Fine! I like it a lot better not so blooming hot!"

Patty looked up suddenly, for the lapse into slang made her think that the pastry cook had been on her guard at lunch time, and had now fallen back to what must be her usual diction.

The old lady was smiling, and as she took her cup and sat down near the girls, Patty felt a sudden aversion.

But she reproached herself for such a feeling toward one who had not only been kind and polite but had helped them out of a real predicament.

By way of salving her conscience, she assumed a kinder manner, and gently readjusted the fur stole.

A Queer Chaperon

"What a dear girl you are!" said Mrs. Doremus, in a burst of admiration. "I don't wonder Little Billee loves you."

Patty stared at her in astonishment.

"You do know Captain Farnsworth, then!" she exclaimed, "or how would you know he is called that by his intimate friends?"

The chaperon looked confused.

"I think I have heard you call him that since you've been here."

"Indeed you haven't! I never speak of him that way to strangers!"

"Come, come, Patty, don't get wrathy!" said Philip, smiling at the lifted chin and tossed head.

"No, I won't," and Patty realised her own foolishness. "Forgive me, Mrs. Doremus, I suppose I'm a silly young thing. But you see, I've never been engaged before and I'm a little fussy about it!"

"Oh, that's all right, young folks ought to be like that. My, when I was engaged, I flew off my head if anybody so much as looked at my young man!"

"It couldn't have been so very long ago," smiled Patty, who had suddenly come to the conclusion that Mrs. Doremus was not so very old, and was, doubtless, prematurely grey-haired.

"Oh yes, many and many a year. But memory is still green, and the sight of young lovers makes my mind turn back, as to a well-remembered page."

Again, Patty caught the strange inflection, as if Mrs. Doremus' words were not quite sincere.

"Come, girls," said Philip, "as you've finished your coffee, let's be thinking about starting."

"I don't want to go!" protested Helen; "it's perfectly lovely here, and we can just as well stay an hour longer as not. Can't we, Mr. Herron?"

"So far as I am concerned, yes. But, unless you start soon, you may find the roads impassable, and be obliged to remain here over night."

"Oh, I've the idea!" Helen cried, "you men go back to town, and leave us girls here to stay the night with Mrs. Doremus! I do think that would be fine! You'd take care of us, wouldn't you?"

She turned her bright, coaxing face to the apple-cheeked old lady, with mute appeal.

To her surprise, Mrs. Doremus was suddenly

afflicted with a hard coughing spell. She choked and nearly strangled, growing red in the face, and gasping for breath.

Herron jumped up and quickly led her from the room, with some hasty words about fresh air.

Van Reypen looked angry and a bit puzzled, but Patty was deeply concerned for the old lady's comfort.

"Let me go, too," she exclaimed, rising, "she needs me,—not Mr. Herron."

"Sit down, Patty," Philip ordered, somewhat gruffly. "Stay where you are. There are plenty of women servants to look after her."

"But she's so nice, Phil! Too nice to have only servants' care."

"Sit down, I tell you. You can't go to her. Remember, Patty, you're not a member of this Club."

"Oh, that's so," and Patty sat down.

"All right," said Herron, returning; "she just choked a little, that's all. And she has chronic throat trouble, so it rather strangled her. She sends you her adieux, and begs to be excused from further appearance."

"Why, of course," said Patty, "she mustn't think of returning. And we're going now, anyhow. Stop your nonsense, Helen, and come, let's get our coats."

" Don't wanna! "

" I know you don't, you old goose, but you must." Patty took her cousin's arm and led her off to the cloak-room.

" Be goody-girl," Herron called after her, " and we'll stop at any place you like for afternoon tea."

" Oh, will you? " and Helen brightened up suddenly. " At the Sunset Tea-room? "

" Yes, wherever you say."

The sleigh came to the door,—horses prancing, bells jingling, and the driver cracking his whip, in true old-time style.

" Oh, wait a minute," Patty cried, as they were about to get in, " where's my stole? Mrs. Doremus still has it! I'm so glad I remembered."

" I'll get it," volunteered Herron. " You others wait here."

He was gone so long that Philip suggested Mrs. Doremus had decamped with the fur.

" Was it valuable, Patty? "

" Yes; that is, it's a perfectly good piece of kolinski."

" Better make up your mind to order another. Something tells me you'll never see that particular animal again."

"How silly, Phil, of course I will. They don't have kleptomaniacs in a Club like this."

"People of acquisitive tendencies are to be found everywhere. However, here comes Herron with the pelt, but he looks as if he'd had to fight for it!"

Sure enough, Herron appeared, greatly ruffled. His face was red, his eyes glowering, and his whole aspect that of a man who has been through a war of words.

"All right," he said, with a very evident effort to seem at ease, "here's your fur cape,—or whatever you call it."

"Stole," corrected Philip.

"No it wasn't!" cried Herron. "Mrs. Doremus had mislaid it, in her excitement, and couldn't remember for the moment where it was. But she found it at once."

He put the fur round Patty's neck, and assisted her into the sleigh in silence.

"Something's up!" that astute young woman remarked to herself. "I must find out about it, —that is, if it concerns me, and I pretty much think it does."

But she was far too canny to ask questions of

Herron then. She chatted gaily and smiled brightly, telling herself the while, that there could be nothing really wrong.

The snow had almost ceased falling, and before they had gone more than a mile, the sun came straggling through the clouds, as it sometimes does when anxious to finish off a snowstorm quickly.

And Helen was delighted, for she knew that meant they would stop at her favourite tearoom, and she could have the chocolate and sweet cakes which were her beloved though " forbidden fruit."

CHAPTER VIII

IN THE TEA-ROOM

THE Sunset Tea-room did not belie its name. The draperies and decorations were of true sunset tints,—gold and amber, with glints of red, and all most harmonious and effective.

The quartette found a pleasant table, where the shaded lights cast a soft glow over the pretty appointments, and Helen picked up the menu card with pleased anticipation.

"You're just incorrigible, Bumble!" laughed Patty; "you promised me you'd cut out sweet things for afternoon tea, yet I see you voraciously devouring the cake list!"

"I know it, Patsy Poppet, but today is an exception,——"

"What day isn't? All right, girlie, but like Lady Jane in the play 'there will be too much of you in the coming by-and-by!'"

"There can't be too much of a good thing!" said Herron, gaily, "so go ahead, Miss Barlow, choose all the puff paste and whipped cream you want."

"If I did that, I'd order the whole card," Helen returned, "and that wouldn't do at all."

"Like the story of the little pickaninny," put in Van Reypen; "they said he was ill from eating too much watermelon. And a neighbour said, 'Law sakes! Dey ain't no such t'ing as too much watermillion!' and the reply was, 'Den dere wasn't enough boy!'"

"That's it exactly," and Helen smiled; "there aren't too many kinds of cakes here,—but there isn't quite enough me!"

But after some careful consideration, she selected the most irresistible dainties, and the others also made their choice.

"You never told us the 'Eagle' story," Herron reminded, as they waited for their order to be served.

"That's so," said Patty, "what was it, Helen? Didn't you say it had to do with the end of the war?"

"That's as you look at it. Here's the tale. You see, down at Beverly, just before the close of the Revolution, there appeared a few eagles——"

"Bald?" inquired Phil.

In the Tea-room

"Dunno if they were bald or long-haired or blonde,—but they were eagles,—real, live American eagles. And they had never been seen in that locality before. Well, their appearance heralded the end of the Revolution,—and immediately it ended."

"Great!" cried Philip, a little ironically; "it reminds me of the slave who called out, ' Oh, King live forever!' and *immediately* the King lived forever!"

"I shouldn't wonder if that's a better story than mine," laughed Helen, "but I'll proceed with mine, as, if I don't, I may not get it done before my cakies come. Well, the Revolution ended, and no eagles were seen any more at all, in or near Beverly. Until,—near the close of the Civil War, those same eagles appeared in Beverly again!"

"Sure they were the same ones? Pretty old birds!"

"Oh, eagles live thousands of years! That's *nothing* for an eagle! Anyway, the eagles came, and the Civil War soon came to its close."

"Now then for the point of this tale," said Herron. "Has friend eagle showed up of late?"

"He has!" cried Helen triumphantly; "several eagles were seen there last week! Now, *I* believe this war will soon end!"

"The American eagle is a war-ender, all right!" declared Phil, "and I hope to goodness, Helen, your pet scheme works out. Just how long after the eagles' arrival is peace declared? Usually, I mean."

"That I can't say. Nor do I swear to the truth of the story. But I tell the tale as 'twas told to me, and you can take it or leave it."

"I'll take it," said Patty, promptly. "I'm a wee bit superstitious, and I like to think of the eagles appearing as a harbinger of hope of peace,—like the Ark dove."

"It can't do any harm to believe it," and Philip smiled at her; "and it may do good. If you believed in a thing I'm sure it would make me do so, too, and if a lot of us believe, it might help to make it come true."

"Then we'll all believe," said Helen, "and I'm sure glad to be the means,—in a small way, —of helping my country toward peace!"

"One can scarcely call it *more* than a small way," Herron said, mock-judicially, "and yet it's as much as many of us do. Even if we're willing, we can't perform. I'm ready to fly to

[124]

the ends of the earth for my old Uncle Sam, but I have to await orders."

" And I can't help feeling glad that you do," interposed Helen. " What would us girls do without you boys to play with? To be sure, we'll give you up

" When it's ' Ready! Fire! ' and you fire away,
 And fight 'em to a finish for the U. S. A."

" For us, it's ' Ready! Fly! ' and we fly away," and Philip looked eager at the thought. " I hate to leave my ain fireside, and that of friends and fellow citizens, but there is an urge——"

" You sound like Sam Blaney! " and Patty laughed. " He was always talking about the Cosmic Urge."

" That isn't in it with the Urge of the Flag. Oh, you girls don't know the *thrill* of feeling that you can be of real help,—however small or insignificant help it is! "

Patty gave Phil an admiring glance. She liked this sort of talk and though she knew of his patriotism, she had rarely heard him express it so strongly.

" Here's your cakaroons! " cried Herron, as

the tray appeared, and the tea and chocolate were served to them.

"Now, no war talk, for the moment," begged Helen. "It does interfere with my enjoyment of my frugal fare, to get stirred up, even by patriotism."

"Let's talk about our visit at the Club," said Patty, suddenly. "Did it strike any of you that Mrs. Doremus was a very strange person?"

"Did it!" said Philip, with emphasis. "Well, *rather!*"

"As how?" asked Herron.

"To begin with, she was no lady," Van Reypen asserted.

"Just what do you mean?" pursued Herron.

"That's a little harsh," Patty demurred, "but she certainly acted queer."

"What do you care?" Herron demanded, "she served the purpose of chaperon, when no one else was there to do so."

"Yes, I know. The principal thing I noticed that seemed strange was that she didn't knit!"

"My goodness gracious! I never thought of that!" exclaimed Herron.

"Perhaps she couldn't," laughed Patty.

"At least, she could have made a stab at it,

which is what most women do. Oh, you
needn't laugh! I've observed them! They
spend more time holding their work off and
looking at it, or counting stitches, or picking
back—whatever that is!—or correcting mis-
takes, or, just patting and pinching the thing!"

"You're right, Mr. Herron," and Patty
laughed at his graphic description, which was
greatly aided by his dramatic imitation of a
nervous knitter. "But Mrs. Doremus didn't
even do that. Nor did she say anything about
it,—which was queer, I think."

"Yes, it was queer," agreed Helen, "though
I hadn't thought of it before. Oh, Patty!
This cream cake is a *dream!*"

"A dream cake?" suggested Philip, "a cream
cake dream cake,—well, what I noticed especially about our friend and benefactor, was her
shoes."

Herron looked up quickly.

"No lady would wear shoes like those!" Van
Reypen asserted.

"I didn't see them," said Patty, "her dress
was so long. Queer, to have such very long
skirts, nowadays."

"No lady would wear such a long skirt," Van
Reypen went on.

"Oh, Phil, don't be so critical," and Patty shook her head at him. "Mrs. Doremus wasn't fashionable, I know, nor even very well posted as to a chaperon's duties, but she was kind, and she filled what I think is known as a long-felt want."

"She told me something you haven't told me, Patty," and Helen looked reproachfully at her cousin.

"What?"

"She says your Big Bill is coming to New York in February."

"She did! A lot she knows about it! She's a meddlesome Matty,—I think! And, besides, he isn't,—'cause why? 'cause if he had been he would have told his little Patty person!"

"How'd she know?" asked Philip.

"Dunno. She may have heard some rumours or had inside information from somebody. I thought you'd be glad to hear it, Patty."

"I am, if it's true. But, I never believe good news, till I'm pretty positive. It saves disappointment, lots of times."

"Little philosopher!" and Van Reypen gave her a sympathetic glance. "But I shouldn't be surprised if that news were true, for I saw something in the paper this morning that looked like it."

"When I get home, I'll have a letter," and Patty blushed a little, "and I rather guess I'll be told, if there's anything to tell."

"Of course you will," said Herron. "Also, I'd not be surprised if Miss Fairfield knows more herself than she tells! These letters from Washington to personal friends are not to be read aloud in the market-place,—for more reasons than one."

Patty looked conscious, but said nothing. Indeed, it was true that Farnsworth often wrote bits of comment on subjects that Patty knew must not be talked over nor his information divulged. And so, she preserved a scrupulous secrecy regarding any war news her letters might hold.

Also, once in a while, Farnsworth sent Patty a little letter, sealed and enclosed in another. This he sometimes asked her not to open until a certain time, or he asked her to mail it in New York, for secret reasons.

All of these matters Patty attended to with punctilious care and she loved to think that she was helping her Little Billee and also her country.

"One doesn't read one's love letters aloud,
—naturally!" and Patty looked down and
blushed.

"Of course not!" cried Helen; "I should
say *not!* And especially yours! Oh, I know!
You've read bits to me now and then, and if
what you *omit* is any more—ahem—well,
turtle-dovish than what you *do* read, and I've
no doubt it *is*——"

"It is," Patty returned, with unmoved equanimity. "What's the use of being engaged if
one may not be what you call turtle-dovey!
I'm not a bit embarrassed about it. But for
my part, I think Mrs. Doremus was decidedly
over-curious and forward about me and my
affairs."

"Unladylike," put in Van Reypen.

"How you harp on that word!" exclaimed
Patty. "I don't think it was so much that, as
a lack of good breeding——"

"Oh, come now, Patty, didn't you catch on?"

"Catch on to what?"

"Why, that Mrs. Doremus was no lady,—
because,—she was a man."

"What!"

"She sure was! And I'd like an explanation,
Herron. I thought I'd let the matter pass

until I could see you alone, but I think it's better to have it out here and now. You brought that person to us, you fixed up the matter, now tell us about it."

George Herron burst into laughter.

" I own up! " he confessed, " I did it! Alone I did it! Oh, it *was* a joke! "

Patty looked puzzled. " A man? " she said; " masquerading? "

" Just that, dear lady," and Herron laughed afresh. " I couldn't help it! There was no woman on the premises save the housekeeper's daughter, who was only a girl of fifteen or so. There was no way to keep you girls there for luncheon except by providing a chaperon. So, —I did my best. Don't look so shocked. It was only a harmless jest. Surely, the quondam chaperon was in no way objectionable; and, as Miss Fairfield admits, she—or he— filled a long-felt want! "

" But who was she—or he? "

" One of the Club attendants. He's on the house force, sort of manager of the heating and electricity departments. Well, I was put to it, as you know, and I was asking him what to do, and he suggested,—or to be accurate, he fell in with my suggestion,—that he slip into one of the housekeeper's gowns and play 'Charley's Aunt.' So he did."

"What do you mean, 'Charley's Aunt'?" asked Helen.

"That's an old play, all college chaps know, where a young man played chaperon just as Munson did today. Not going to be mad about it, are you, Miss Fairfield?"

"Of course she isn't!" cried Helen; "I think it's a great joke! And, as you say, we couldn't have stayed there, otherwise! Oh, Patty, don't get on your Puritanic high horse! It was only a regard for a convention, anyway, and the convention was regarded!"

Helen went off in peals of laughter at the reminiscence of the so-called chaperon. "No wonder he wore a long skirt! To cover up his feet,—of course! And his white wig! Oh, it was perfect! Where did he get a wig so handy?"

"It was in a little room where a lot of things are, left, I believe, from some theatrical jinks. Anyway, he said he could make up perfectly, —and he did."

"Oh, he did! I think he was fine!"

"He was fine, Helen, as a masquerader," said Patty, slowly, "but I don't think it was a fine performance,—by any means!" She looked gravely at Herron, who reddened a little, but stood his ground.

"Oh, come, now, Miss Fairfield, I didn't mean any harm. Honest, I never dreamed of offending you, or annoying you,—I thought only of how to manage to keep you there for our little party. Moreover I thought you'd think it a great joke,—honest, I did."

Herron's clear brown eyes were so earnest and his expression so troubled, that Patty's heart was touched.

"I don't doubt it, Mr. Herron," and she smiled kindly at him, "but it wasn't just the thing to do,—was it, Phil?"

"Oh, well, forget it, Pattibelle, and if you can't forget it—forgive it, anyway. Herron meant no harm and I knew at once, that Dame Doremus,—as I told you,—was no lady! But I saw through Herron's motive as well as his joke, and there's no great harm done that I can see."

"I agree with Phil," and Helen nodded her head positively; "I'm jolly glad you did it, for otherwise, I'd have had to come home without any luncheon!"

"Than which there could be no worse hardship!" Herron sympathised. "Am I forgiven, Miss Fairfield?"

"I'm not sure," Patty gave him a half smile, "I'll think it over. Didn't you know this man?"

"Not from Adam! But, you know, you can size up a chap a lot from appearances, and he was a good sort, and amenable to—well, to argument."

"Golden argument," laughed Philip. "You put it over, all right, Herron, old chap, and I'm sure Miss Fairfield will overlook her chaperon's extra-sized feet! Had it not been that I noticed those, I might have been fooled myself. For the boy,—isn't he a boy?"

"About twenty-five or so,—I should judge."

"Well, his face was boyish, and his general effect young, yet he donned age with his wig and gown, and on the whole I call it a remarkable bit of disguise."

"No wonder he didn't knit!" exclaimed Helen. "And no wonder he choked when I proposed that we girls stay there longer!"

"He acted queerly all the time;" Patty looked thoughtful. "I'm thinking he knew too much about me and my affairs."

"What are you getting at now, Patty?"

In the Tea-room

Helen asked. "Think he'll reappear in his proper person, and presume on our acquaintance?"

"No," said Patty, "I'm afraid he *won't!*"

Van Reypen looked at her.

"Of course, the chap's all right, eh, Herron? Credentials, and that?"

"Must be or they wouldn't have him in the Club."

"There are spies everywhere," said Patty, in a whisper.

"Oh, Pitty-Pat!" cried Helen, "is *that* what's troubling you? Well, well! Those letters you get from Washington do sure go to your head! I see it, now, people! Bill tells Patty to look out for spies, and so,—she sees them everywhere!"

"Spies in the brooks, spies in the pastry-cooks!" exclaimed Herron, and Helen giggled.

"Yes, and I shouldn't wonder if Patty suspects every one of us!"

"You needn't laugh," and Patty shook her curly head. "There *is* danger, isn't there, Phil?"

"Of course, child. But even if this bad Mrs. Doremus was a spy,—she learned nothing from us, today."

[135]

" She—he asked a heap of questions."

" But nothing of any importance. It seems to me that,—Munson, is that his name?—only showed such curiosity as would become an elderly lady talking with two charming girls. You practically told her—him,—of your engagement, Patty, so you mustn't wonder that he showed some interest."

" I s'pose so. Well, we won't say anything more about it. I'm foolish, I suppose,—but I don't like that sort of thing."

" Then I apologise," said Herron, heartily; " I'm truly sorry I did it, but I ask you to believe that I would not have done it, had it occurred to me for a moment that you would feel about it as you do."

" I do believe that," and Patty's blue eyes shone with forgiveness and understanding. " I know, Mr. Herron, that you really did it out of the kindest motives, and I exonerate you——"

" Wow! what a big word! " cried Helen. " If you're exonerated, Mr. Herron, surely you can't ask for more! Why, I thought to be ex— what do you call it? was what the Pope does! "

" No, my child, that's to be excommunicated, and Mr. Herron shan't be that! " And Patty beamed full forgiveness on the culprit.

CHAPTER IX

CAPTAIN WILLIAM FARNS-WORTH sat in his room, opening his morning mail. Or rather, his morning mail was waiting to be opened, while he eagerly perused a letter from Miss Patricia Fairfield.

"For the love of pickled peppers!" he exclaimed, in a self-addressed murmur, "she *didn't!* she *couldn't!*"

For the letter said,—in part:

"I am *so* glad you're thinking of coming to New York in February! That's soon here! Which day? What hour? Oh, my Little Billee, how can I *wait* to see you! I want to look in those dear, big, loving blue eyes, and have them answer the questions I want to ask. You know what the questions are! Oh, well, suppose I do know the answers,—I guess a little Patty Blossom can ask over again if her big Sir Galahad loves her,—and why,—and how much, —and a few such things,—that are important, if true! And there is nothing in this whole

[137]

round world truer than our love,—is there, dear? I just *live* in it,—when I am alone, I thing of nothing but US, and, I'm afraid I am absent-minded, even when other people are about. Do come home soon,—come to your own Patty Posy. Tell me quick *when* to look for you! Why didn't you tell me sooner there was hope of seeing you soon? My own dear big man, my own, my owner, my ownest, I'm now and forever

"Your

"PATTY BLOSSOM."

Farnsworth frowned,—he looked puzzled, amazed, hurt.

Again he resorted to expletives. "Great jumping kangaroos!" he said to himself, "I can't see it! Patty never did such a thing! never! But if not, how did she know? I believe the very walls have not only ears but tongues and pens in their hands, and a whole wireless outfit beside! I *can't* suspect Patty,— and yet,—all women are curious,—and, of course, this doesn't matter so much,—but if I can't trust her in everything how can I trust her at all?"

With a sigh, he laid the letter aside, **and** turned to his business correspondence.

Letters

Farnsworth's position was a responsible one, and it contained and involved many secrets that must be carefully guarded. Among these was the fact and date of his next trip to New York. It was on a matter of moment, and it was not desirable that his absence from Washington should be known. He had written Patty about it, but he had enclosed the message in a sealed envelope, with directions not to open it until he wired her to do so. Thus, he planned, she would know it in time, but the information could not leak out. And now it had leaked out. Patty knew and made no secret of the knowledge that he was expected in New York. Had she told others? And,—worst of all,—had she opened the sealed letter before he told her to? This was incredible,—yet, what other solution or theory was possible? And there was to be considered a grouchy old Colonel, who would make all sorts of trouble for Captain Farnsworth if it became known that he was careless with his personal correspondence.

Because of his well-trained mind, and his power of concentration, Farnsworth forced himself to attend to matters in hand, but ever and again flashed across his preoccupied brain the fact that Patty had disregarded his instructions.

He lived with a pleasant family in the Capital, and his quarters were the whole of the second floor of the small house. This gave him a good-sized sitting room, which was his private office, and here he transacted all business that didn't require his presence at the more public buildings.

He kept doggedly at work, determined not to let the disturbing episode interfere with his efficiency. And he succeeded, but only by dint of perseverance in his resolve not to think of Patty at all.

This was difficult, for every glance of his eye fell on something remindful of her. A photograph on his desk; other little snapshots lurking among his papers; a paper-cutter she had given him; indeed, the pen he wrote with was her parting gift; and all spoke eloquently of the girl he had so reluctantly left behind him.

"Busy, Captain?" called a gay voice, and a merry face peeped in at the door.

"Always busy," he returned, cheerily, "but never too busy to say good morning."

"Oh, I know what that means! That I must

say good morning, and nothing more! But I do want just half a dozen more words."

The piquant face smiled coaxingly, as Lena Richards danced in. She was the daughter of the house, a dark-haired, olive-skinned little gipsy, who, being quite spoiled by her doting parents, assumed the right to have her own way with every one else.

Farnsworth liked her as no one could help doing, but he was often obliged to speak more curtly than he liked to, or she would intrude too often on his time.

She wore a smock of pink linen and her curly hair was bundled into a little Dutch cap. She came in, with the venturesome air of a mischievous child, and perched saucily on the corner of the big desk.

"You see," she began, "I'm in an awful scrape—well, that is, *I'm* not, but somebody else is——"

"Who isn't?" said Farnsworth, smiling at the roguish little face that wore such a troubled frown.

"Yes, I s'pose everybody is, more or less, from the President down. And when you think of that, my little brother does seem small, but—you see, to me——"

" It's a national calamity? "

" Personal rather than national,—yet it may be said to be international."

" Many of our troubles are. Your story interests me strangely,—my che-ild,—but truly, Lena, I can't take time now to hear the yarn. I suppose your fudge was lumpy, or your new ribbons don't match your frock,—is that it? "

" You always talk as if I were a child! " and the scarlet lips pouted petulantly.

" Of course! I always think of you as a kiddy in a middy."

" This isn't a middy, it's a smock, and a very grown up one at that."

" Do smocks grow up? Thought they only grew old. Well, anyway, whatever your age, I've no time to waste on you this morning. My country needs me! "

" You're always so unkind to me,——" and two crystal drops formed in the big, brown eyes.

Now, William Farnsworth was the sort of man who can't stand seeing a woman in distress. And though he knew that this sixteen-year-old chit could have no real or deep trouble, he yet could not bring himself to speak sternly to her, and tell her to leave the room.

Letters

Against his will, he obeyed the dictates of his kind heart, and taking out his watch, said:

"I'll give you ten minutes. Spill your story in Papa's ear!"

The dark little face lighted with gladness, and Lena murmured, "How good you are! Listen, then! You know my friend, Gracie Hadley?"

"Haven't the pleasure. Who's she in America?"

"Well, she's just Gracie, that's all. And—sh!"—Lena looked cautiously about, "don't breathe it, but she's in love with an English chap who's over here. And her mother doesn't approve——"

"Why? Who's the Britisher?"

"I don't want to tell you, 'cause it's Gracie's secret——"

"All right; I don't want to know anyway. But where do I come in? I hate to hurry you, but I'm assuming I play a part in this tragedy, and I want my cue, for honest to goodness, Lena, I've troubles of my own!"

"Yes, I know, Captain, and I won't be but a minute explaining. Well, Gracie has been corresponding with this man,——"

"Oh, naughty! naughty!"

"Hush! It's all right; only of course, she doesn't want her mother to know. Well, she tears up his letters, but—*what* do you think!"

"Censor?"

"No! but the man has given her her letters to him——"

"Returned them!"

"No; I mean yes,—but for this reason—you fluster me so,—with your snapping up!"

"Well, well, go and tell it in your own way. But, for Heaven's sake, hurry up!"

"All right. You see he gave her these letters to save for him just while he's away somewhere, and he wants them when he comes back."

"Can't she write some more?"

"Oh! You're so unfeeling! So—why, you're *stupid!*"

"Pardon,—sorry! Fire away."

"Never mind details,—Gracie can't keep them at home, for fear her mother will find them—she snoops awfully! And—*I* can't keep them here,——"

"For a similar reason?"

"Yes; exactly! So,—Captain Farnsworth,— nice, dear Captain Farnsworth, won't you let me hid them in here,—among your things?"

"Goodness! Little One, is that all you want?

Letters

Sure! Hide them wherever you like in my domain. Your eagle-eyed mother won't find them in here! But, hold on! Nothing that wouldn't get by the Censor, is there?"

"Oh, goodness, no! Nothing like that!"

"Guess I'll have to have a glimpse of 'em, though. Not to pry into the lovers' confidences, of course, but because I can't harbour papers unless I'm satisfied of their contents."

"All right,—that goes! I'll get them now;" and running from the room, Lena returned with a small packet of letters tied with blue ribbon.

Farnsworth examined the envelopes, and glanced here and there at the written pages.

"All right," he said, re-tying the packet, "internal evidence proves conclusively to *my* mind that these documents are just what you describe them to be. Say we put them in the top drawer of my chiffonier; how's that?"

"Fine! Mother would never dream of looking in your room!"

"I should hope not! And now may I, without undue haste, bid you a very good morning?"

"S'pose I've *got* to go, if you put it like that. I did want to tell you more about Gracie; and there's something I want to ask you."

"Not now, not now, my child. I am busy—see? B-U-S-Y! My Flag comes before my friends! Thus, you see my friends follow the Flag!"

"You are so witty! And so kind. Thank you lots, Captain, and when you're not so busy, may I talk to you again?"

"If that time ever comes! But it never will unless you clear out! Scoot now!" Farnsworth held the door persuadingly open, and Lena didn't scoot, but she went slowly and reluctantly out.

"The pretty little nuisance!" muttered the Captain, as he closed and locked his door.

Without further interruption, Bill put in the morning on his war work, and at last was free to consider the case against Patty Fairfield.

"She's true blue," he thought, "far too true to do anything she deemed wrong or even indiscreet. But I suppose she didn't realise how definite,—how imperative my instructions were, —maybe I didn't tell her distinctly enough,— maybe she forgot,—or was really overcome with a desire to know what was in that sealed note. Oh, well, I must warn her further. I hate to hurt her,—I can't let her think I distrust her,—and Lord knows I *don't!* How I

wish I had more time! But I've that appointment at two—and—whew! I'll have to
scribble to Patty pretty fast, whatever I say!"

The result, after one or two torn-up attempts,
was this:

" My Own Patty Blossom,—my Posy Face,—
my Best Beloved: I've only a minute to write
this time, and so I must come to the point at
once. Dear Heart,—*did* you open the sealed
note before I told you to? Oh, well,—I know
you did so never mind about that,—but, my
precious little girl, don't, *please* don't ever do it
again. You see, I send you notes thus, so that
you can open them in haste when I wire you
that you may. Now, if you open them sooner,
I never know where we stand. In this matter,
darling, please consider my wishes—and, especially because I meant to send a really valuable
paper to you, in order that you might hand it
to me when I do come to New York, and I
won't have to carry it with me or trust it to the
general mail. I can't explain all these matters,
as you know, dear, but I do want to feel that
in the government work that is entrusted to
me, I can as implicitly trust *you* to be my aid
and helper. Can't I, Sweetheart? Of course,
I know I can, and I know your eager haste to

learn my plans led you to open that letter before time. So, don't do it again, and all will
be well. Now, I've not another minute, but I
must take time to say once again that I love
you, and you're all the world to me, my dear,
dear little Posy Patty.

" And I'm your faithful and devoted
" LITTLE BILLEE."

When Patty received this letter she read it
and sat aghast. What could he mean? She
had never opened a letter until he told her to!
Many times she had received permission by
mail or by wire, and then she had opened the
sealed notes so frequently enclosed in Bill's
letters to her. But never before she got the
word! Never,—never!

Again she read the pages from Washington.
Had Farnsworth imagined it or what had made
him dream that she had done such a thing?

She? Not to be trusted! When every
thought she had, every deed she did was with
the one trust and hope that she might help her
Captain,—even in the smallest way!

She went to her writing desk and from a
locked drawer she took Bill's sealed note, that
had come with a recent letter.

It was still sealed. Why would he think she

[148]

had opened it? Oh, well, she thought, something has made him think so. I must write him at once that I didn't. He'll believe me, of course. I know his faith and trust, and they are not misplaced, that's certain!

So, a letter was quickly written and despatched telling the Captain that his aid and helper in New York had not been false to her trust in the minutest particular.

But Patty was still puzzled and gave much thought to the matter.

When Van Reypen came to say good-bye on the eve of his departure for camp, he found a quiet and worried little girl, who received him with but a slight smile.

"Well, my Lady Fair, you look as if you'd lost your last friend,—or, perhaps, as if you were about to lose him! May I take this general air of gloom as a tribute to my regrettable absence? Is it just 'cause you're going to lose your little old friend that you look so disconsolate?"

"No, sir! it isn't! In the first place, I don't look sad, and in the second place, if I do, it isn't because I'm doing any 'Leah, the forsaken,' act! I shall miss you, of course, but in these days we must learn to miss people!"

"That's true, Patty, and have you any idea,
—any faint glimmering of a notion, how I shall
miss you?"

"Phil, I know all grades of missing! I'm no
novice at it. Since this war called them, I've
missed acquaintances, casual friends, old
friends, relatives, and, of course, most of all,
my own Little Billee. Now, I shall miss you,
—and I know you'll miss me,—but, you'll soon
get so interested in your work—in the great
game,—that you'll—oh, not forget me, I'm
sure,—but my memory will become, let us say,
a little blurred."

"Indeed it won't! But, hold on here, if it
isn't my departure, what is it that has made
your countenance sicklied o'er with a pale cast
of—something or other?"

"Rice powder, probably! Does it really
make me look sickly? Good gracious!" Patty
scrubbed at her cheeks with her handkerchief,
until they were rosy indeed.

"Nope; you can't rub it off! It's ingrained.
Come now, what's up?"

"Well, I am bothered. Philip, how do war
secrets leak out?"

"How do they keep from it, you mean!
Why, Patty, the end and aim of a majority of

our citizens seems to be to chatter and make trouble thereby. What's exploded now?"

"Nothing that I can tell you,—only,—well,—never mind."

"You transparent little goose! Have you been and went and told something Farnsworth told you not to?"

"No, I haven't! But he thought I did, so it's just as bad!"

"No; not *just* as bad,—but, bad. What was it?"

"Never mind, but he thought I opened a sealed envelope and it's still sealed."

"Has it been out of your possession?"

"Not for a minute!"

"Good! and locked away when you are asleep?"

"Always; locked in a secret drawer."

"Good, again. Then, you're all right. But let me warn you, Patty, to be most exceedingly cautious. Farnsworth's work is of the highest importance, and his plans must not be known in advance. I know this even better than you do, and I beg of you to be even over-careful of any orders he may give you."

"Oh, I am! I do! But you see, this matter must have leaked out some other way, and he thought it was because of my knowledge of it."

"Patty!" Philip spoke suddenly; "did you have that letter with you that day at the Timothy Grass Club?"

"Yes; I had just received it that morning."

"Where did you carry it?"

"In my fur stole; there's a buttoned pocket in the end of it, and it's a safe place."

"And that Munson,—that masquerader,—wore your stole!"

"So he did!" and Patty looked frightened. "But, no! that's all right, Phil. The enclosed note was still sealed when I reached home, and it is sealed yet!"

"Very well; but don't take any chances. Leave your letters at home and carefully locked up, if they contain anything outside your entirely personal affairs. I speak whereof I know, Patty, and you *must* be careful!"

"I will, Philip, oh, truly I will," and Patty gave the promise in all sincerity.

CHAPTER X

A VALENTINE

"WELL," said Helen Barlow, dashing into Patty's room one morning, "I am certainly having the time of my sweet young life! They may say what they like about the horrors of war, and there are plenty of them, and nobody knows that better than I do, and nobody does more to help our side than you do, but all the same, my fairy-fair cousin, I do get a lot of pleasant parties and happy hours out of it all."

"Why, Bumble-Bee, what's up now?"

"Look at all these letters in my morning's mail! And nearly every one an invitation to a gathering of some sort, connected with Our Boys. Dinners and evening parties and little dances, all for the Khaki and the Blue! Red Cross Benefits, private charities and any number of War Relief meetings! Don't think I'm a heartless wretch, Patsy, but I do love the everlasting gadding about, and meeting people and being in the excitement of it all!"

[153]

"Good for you, Bumble," said Nan, coming in, "having heard your views, I'll invite you to help me with a small and early bazaar I'm arranging for a Valentine fête."

"Of course I'll do all I can, Nan. Tell me more. When is it to be?"

"On the twelfth; we want to sell valentines to send to the soldiers in camp, and incidentally, have a good time, and, moreover, make a little money for my committee."

"Where you going to have it?" asked Patty, looking up from her desk, where she was writing letters.

"Why, here," said Nan. "You needn't do much, Pattikins, you've so many irons in the fire; Bumble and I will run this show."

"Good for you! I have about all I can manage on a paltry twenty-four hours a day. But I'll buy a valentine of you to send to my own particular Soldier Boy. Oh, Nan, isn't he the dearest thing! Just look at this new picture of him! Did anybody *ever* look so well in a uniform?"

"He is sure great!" exclaimed Bumble, taking the picture; "I don't wonder you rave over him, Patty."

"Nor I," Nan agreed. "He's so big, yet so

A Valentine

well-proportioned that he doesn't look *too* big."

"Oh, *thank* you, Nan! I dunno what I'd do if he were *too* big!" Patty showed mock alarm at the thought. "You see, the bigger he is the smaller I seem, but I'm trying to emulate Bumble, and get a little more weighty. It's hard, though, with the food conservation to be looked after, and the sweetless days here and there——"

"*You* don't have any sweetless days, if you read those long letters you get," put in Helen.

"And pray, how do *you* know as to their sweetness?"

"Oh, I'm a mind reader, and when I see you peruse a letter, and fairly lap it up, like a cat, and then sit looking like the cat who ate the canary, I don't have to be a detective to deduce that the letter was a sweet one!"

"Good for you, Bumble! You guessed right the very first time! My Captain's letters *are* sweet, and so is he!"

"Sounds like a valentine! And he's in love and so is she!"

"We are," said Patty, complacently. "And that's no secret. As to valentines, pick me out the prettiest and the wittiest and the one that reads best, and save it for me, when you two busy bees have this festa,—or whatever you call it."

"That's so! What shall we call it?" and Helen turned to Nan. "Ought to begin with a V. Valentine Valley? Valentine Villa?"

"Not very good," Nan considered. "How's Valentine Verses?"

"All valentines have verses. Help us out, Patty. Do that much for the cause. Give us a name for our Sale."

"Valentine Vendue," said Patty, without looking up from her writing. Though apparently absorbed in her own affairs she had heard all they said.

"A vendue is an auction," objected Nan.

"Oh, well, it means a sale," Patty defended, "and too, of course, you'll auction off the leftovers, they always do at a sale."

"We might have it all an auction,——" began Nan.

"All right, do," returned Patty, "but run away, kiddies, and make your plans somewhere else, won't you? Miss Fairfield is busy."

"Come on, Bumble, we'll go off and flock by ourselves. And we'll plan such a bee-yutiful party that we'll sell enough valentines for the whole National Army."

"Do they want valentines?" asked Helen as she went off with Nan.

"That doesn't matter, my dear. The thing is for us to sell the valentines, and get the money for the committee; and then, if the sweet missives are never sent, it won't matter. But, yes, I think the boys in camp would be jolly glad to get nice loving valentine verses. They needn't know who sends them, of course."

"I shall put my name on all *I* send. I'd like to get a letter back."

"Your mail is full of such letters already! You're a camp belle, Bumble,—you certainly are!"

"I might make a joke about the camp belles are coming!" laughed Helen, "but I'd scorn to do it!"

"Then don't. Come on, now, and let's make lists and all that."

The night of February twelfth found the Fairfield house bedecked for the Valentine Vendue. Palms and flowers and hearts and darts and ribbon streamers and true-love knots were everywhere. Patty had helped both with advice and with actual work and the result was bewilderingly beautiful. Not only the regulation valentines of lace paper and rhymed lines were for sale, but also small and appropriate gifts, in decorated boxes, fancy bonbonnieres, pots and baskets of flowers and flowering plants, and even jewelled trinkets and curios. For these things had been donated for the cause, and the venders hoped the men would buy them for their sweethearts.

Also there were valentines for the soldiers, and boxes of tobacco and cigarettes, containing sentimental missives.

Nan's committee was a large one, and all had worked diligently until the result was even more gratifying than they had hoped.

Patty and Helen wore effective and appropriate costumes for they loved to " dress up," and this was too good a chance to be lost.

Their short frocks were of white tarlatan, edged with lace, and much befrilled. Garlands of tiny rosebuds decked the skirts, and the bodices were trimmed with blue ribbons and gilt paper hearts. Toy Cupids perched on their shoulders, and love-knots of blue decked their hair.

" Do you expect Lieutenant Herron? " Helen asked, as they awaited the guests.

A Valentine

" Rather ! " returned Patty, " considering he's always about wherever you are."

"Me! It's *you* he hovers over! Don't be coy,—you don't fool your little Bumble bee ! "

" Don't you be a silly ! " laughed Patty; " I've no use for the Herron person. If he's here tonight, I'll take it as a favour if you'll charm him away from my haunts."

" Can't do it," and Helen shrugged her shoulders. " He won't be charmed. More-over, I've a lot of my own particular friends coming, and I'll have my hands full to enter-tain them."

" Nan was right when she called you a camp belle. You're looking sweet tonight, Bumble, and I s'pect some man will buy you for a valen tine. Is Chester coming? "

" I s'pose so. Wish he wasn't! He's such a burr."

" Yes, he does stick to you. I'll take him for a while, and give you some rest. I like Mr. Wilde a whole lot."

The guests began to arrive, and soon the rooms were really crowded. The valentines sold quickly, for those who did not want them bought " for the good of the cause."

Patty-Bride

Lieutenant Herron came early, and as Bumble had predicted, he attached himself to Patty's train of followers.

"Such a clutter of men about you!" he exclaimed, as he sought her side, edging his way through a group of valentine buyers. "I say, Miss Fairfield, let some one else sell these people for a while, and you come and have an ice with me, won't you?"

"I'm not selling the people!" cried Patty, smiling, "I'm selling valentines."

"All the same. But you need a rest. Come along, and take it, and come back to your work refreshed."

Patty was tired, and so she asked some one else to take her place for a while, and sauntered off with Herron.

They found a pleasant table in the supper room, and sat down together.

"I saw your friend Van Reypen yesterday," said Herron, after he had given their order.

"Oh, you did? How is he?"

"Fit as a fiddle, and learning to fly, like a young robin!"

"I thought he'd be an apt pupil. Phil is clever at 'most anything."

"Yes, he is. And he takes to aviation like

a duck to water. What do you hear from your other friend?"

"My other friend! Have I then but one more?"

Patty well knew Lieutenant Herron meant Little Billee, but she was always chary of talking about Farnsworth to anybody.

"Only one that you care for; isn't that so?"

"Oh, no! I care for lots of people, and I care for all our soldiers! How can you think otherwise?"

"Yes, in a sense. But only one you care for especially."

"Naturally. If you mean Captain Farnsworth, and I suppose you do,—most girls care especially for the men they are engaged to."

"Are you really engaged to him?"

"Of course I am! Why do you ask?"

"Oh, nothing."

"Your tone belies your words; what do you mean, Lieutenant?"

Patty's eyes gave an ominous flash that her friends all knew indicated serious indignation, but Herron answered lightly, "Oh, nothing, really. I only happened to hear from a friend, of Farnsworth's infatuation for a little dark-eyed beauty down in Washington."

Patty looked at him, amusedly.

"If you're teasing me, your jest is in poor taste, Lieutenant Herron. If you're in earnest, I refuse to listen to you."

"There, there, don't get huffy! I didn't mean to stir you up! I only heard rumours,— doubtless there's nothing in them."

"Doubtless there isn't,—and, also, doubtless it doesn't concern you, if there is!"

Patty was thoroughly angry at the man's impertinence, but she did not want to do anything so conspicuous as to get up and leave the dining-room, where many small tables were occupied by a merry crowd of guests.

"Not at all! not at all! yet, I can't regret my words, since they have given me an opportunity of seeing you when you are ruffled! Prettier than ever! How blue eyes can flash!"

Suddenly Patty felt a fear of this man. He did not seem to ring true. But her quick-wittedness made her realise that to continue angry, was to make him more amused and interested, so she changed her tactics.

"Any girl's eyes would flash at your insinuations," she said, with a sudden bright smile.

A Valentine

"But now I know you are chaffing, I don't mind."

" And how do you know I'm chaffing? "

" Because your own eyes twinkle so."

As a matter of fact, Herron's eyes were snapping maliciously, but Patty ignored this, and deftly turned the subject.

"When do you go back to the Aviation Field? " she inquired.

" Tomorrow, alas! I had hoped for longer leave, but a new class is to be trained, and I must be on the job."

" I can't help marvelling at the courage and bravery of an aviator. It seems to me that you take your life in your hands ever more desperately and dangerously than those actually at the front."

" In a sense, we do," agreed Herron, a little gravely. " As the darky said, ' If yuh gets killed on the ground, yuh knows where yuh is; but if yuh gets killed up in de air,—where is yuh? ' "

" And so many do get killed."

" Yes, but the proportion continually grows smaller, of course, as we learn more of the art."

" Do you call aviation an art? "

"Yes, an Art with a big A! It's a science as well, to be sure; it's also a mechanical process and—it's largely sheer luck!"

"I'm glad Mr. Van Reypen is doing well. He has a cool head, you know."

"Yes, and that's a great thing. A steady nerve, and mental poise come first in the requirements for a successful flyer. When are you to be married, Miss Fairfield?"

"Good gracious! You take my breath away with your sudden questions. Incidentally, they are a bit rude. Do you ask about such personal matters in your home town?"

Herron had the grace to blush. But he said, slowly, "I suppose I would, if I cared as much to know as I do in this case."

"Why?"

"Why? You know why! You must know! Because I'm over head and ears in love with you, myself! Because, though it would add to my misery to know you're to be married soon, yet it would be a blessed relief to know it would *not* be soon!"

"I cannot see, Lieutenant Herron, that these matters concern you at all," said Patty, icily, and then the look of pained reproach he gave her smote her heart. For Patty was a gentle

A Valentine

soul, and rarely hurt the feelings of anybody. "I think I must ask you to drop this subject and never refer to it again." But she spoke softly, and shook off her air of offended dignity.

"Forgive me," he murmured, "truly I didn't mean to! But I couldn't help it. You're right, it's none of my business, and I apologise. Come, I see you're ready to leave here, let us go and buy a valentine, which you shall send to your betrothed, and then you'll forgive me."

His tone was gay again, and glad that the tension of the situation was relieved, Patty went with him to the valentine tables.

"Here's a dandy!" remarked the pretty girl who was selling them. "New idea, too. Funny and yet clever! Want one?"

Herron took the one offered, and smiled as he read its lines.

"You wouldn't dare send *that* to your fiancé!" he said, laughingly.

Carelessly, Patty glanced at it. It was a well-done little sketch of a lover and his lass, leaning over a rustic stile, in true valentine fashion. Cupids and turtle-doves hovered above, and hearts and darts formed a conventional margin.

The lines read:

[165]

Patty-Bride

"Our love is high as Heaven
  And wide as rolling sea;
The vows cannot be riven
  That bind my love and me.
But should our pledge be broken,
  Or should your love be dead,
Send back this tender token
  And let us never wed."

"Good gracious!" laughed Patty, "what a
woe-begone outlook for such a happy-looking
pair! And I'm sure such a dismal foreboding
could never come true for these rustic swains!
They're a real Strephon and Chloe couple!"
  "All the same, I see you don't take my dare."
  "What dare?"
  "I dare you to send that valentine to Captain
Farnsworth."
  "What! You think I hesitate, lest he return
it to me!" The absurdity of this struck Patty
as very funny, and she laughed outright.
  "Yes, I think so," and Herron laughed, too.
  "How ridiculous you are! Why, I'd just as
lief send that as not!"
  "Go ahead, and do it, then. Prove your
words."
  "Will you buy it for me, at a goodly price?"

A Valentine

" Whatever the saleslady asks."

" All right.   What's the price, Maisie? "

Greatly amused, the gay little sales-girl said,
" Ten dollars, sir."

A little daunted, but true to his word, Herron
paid the price, and took Patty to the library,
where there was a desk made ready for any
who desired to address and despatch their
missives then and there.

Patty wrote Farnsworth's Washington address, and Herron held out his hand for the
envelope.

" I'll mail it as I go home," he said, and
Patty gave it to him.

The whole incident made little impression on
her, for though she didn't particularly admire
the valentine, nor did she care for the so-called
" poetry " on it, yet, at the same time, it meant
an extra ten dollar bill in the coffers of the
committee, and that was well worth while.

Not much later, the Lieutenant said good
night, for, as he stated, he had to leave for his
duties early next morning.

" And I'm sorry if I offended you, Miss Fairfield, and I hope you'll forgive me," he begged.
" But,—well, my only excuse is, the temptation
was too great, and the opportunity was mine,

[167]

so I said more than I intended, and more than I ought."

"All right, Lieutenant, if you didn't mean it, I forgive you."

"I don't say I didn't mean it,—for that wouldn't be true; but I didn't mean to tell you of it."

"Then," and Patty spoke gravely, now, "never let any circumstance or opportunity tempt you to do it again."

"Then I mustn't see you," Herron said, in a low voice.

"Very well, then don't see me. It will be far better for both. Where is your sense of honour? of fairness? Another man's fiancée is not to be thought of, save with respect and courtesy."

"I know it," and the man looked miserably sad; "and I do mean to treat you with all respect and courtesy,—but, oh, Miss Fairfield, Patty,—let me call you that just once,—if you knew how broken up I am over it all!"

"Then," said Patty, firmly, though she was touched at the sight of his evident suffering, "then the only thing is for us not to meet again, at all. I'm sorry, Lieutenant Herron, for I like you, but these matters are often out-

side our own will, and so, I can see no way but
for us to keep apart."

"May I not come to see you next time I'm
in town?"

"I think not," said Patty, gently, and then
she bade him a courteous but definite and final
good night.

CHAPTER XI

PATTY'S bedroom was a pretty, cheery and charming place. The sunlight came in through delicate, lacy curtains, the furniture and appointments were all that a fastidious taste could desire, and the pictures and trinkets scattered about were beautiful and attractive. There were always fresh flowers in the vases and the whole effect was conducive to happiness and contentment.

Yet across the lace-covered bed was the outstretched form of somebody who had flung herself there in a very abandonment of woe. Somebody with golden curly hair, from which the boudoir cap had fallen unheeded; somebody who was digging a little wet mop of a handkerchief into eyes that flowed with tears like a very freshet of rain. Somebody who was shaking and quivering with great racking sobs that were all the more agonising because they were silent.

Patty In Tears

Patty was crying. And with her ever-active efficiency, she was making a thorough and complete success of it. Now and then, she would pause, sit up and vigorously wipe her eyes, then she would fling herself back into the nest of damp pillows and start all over again. Her pretty negligée of light blue silk was crumpled into a shocking state; one little slipper had fallen off, and though her face was buried in the pillows her heaving shoulders and tumbled curls still bore witness to the woe that was torturing her soul.

Suddenly, she became angry, and sat up straight, fists clenched, eyes blazing,—fairly gritting her teeth in a wave of indignation.

Then again, grief, deep, hopeless grief overcame her, and back she fell, fresh tears welling up and spilling over.

"Patty," cried Bumble, bouncing into the room, "I've a splendid plan! Let's get a whole lot of top balloons, and—for the love of Michaelovitch Paderewski! what *is* the matter?"

Curiously Bumble looked at the shaking figure on the bed. With a frightened face, she came cautiously toward Patty, unable to believe her eyes at the sight of her cousin's attitude.

"Get out! go 'way!" wailed Patty, in such hollow tones that they scarce seemed her own at all.

"Patty! dear! my own little darling cousin—what *is* it? Tell Bumble! Tell me, dear."

"N-nothing! Go away, I tell you."

"I won't go away! How can I, when I don't know what's the matter with you! Are you ill?"

"No—no—oh, Bumble, don't pester me!"

"But what ails you, Patty? You don't even speak like yourself. I'm going to call Nan."

"No, don't! Yes, do! Oh, I don't care what you do!" and a brand-new deluge poured forth, as Patty sat up and stared at Helen with eyes full of utter woe as well as gushing tears.

Thoroughly frightened, Helen did call Nan, who came at once.

"Why, you poor little thing," she said, sitting down beside Patty, and caressing her, as she offered a fresh handkerchief in place of the squeezed up mop in Patty's hand.

"Never mind, dear, don't try to talk,—just be quiet. And cry all you like,—but, gracious! I didn't know one person *could* hold so many tears! Now, hush, dear, don't talk. Keep right on crying, it'll do you good."

[172]

Patty In Tears

Nan's comforting voice and her tender whimsicality, helped Patty, and she sobbed in Nan's arms, for a time, then, by degrees, her tears began to be somewhat checked, and she stopped shaking.

Nan only patted her gently, and crooned comforting little sounds, that soothed the tortured nerves by their loving tone.

At last, Patty stopped crying for the simple reason, apparently, that her tears had at last become exhausted.

Helen had brought a fresh relay of handkerchiefs, and as Patty half-unconsciously accepted one after another, the bed was strewn with the moistened squares of linen.

"Hold on," warned Bumble, "if you're going to begin again, go easy on this; it's the last one of mine."

"I've plenty," assured Nan, "cry away, Patty, if you like."

Nan's intuition told her that Patty must have her cry out, before any explanation could be forthcoming. And it was so. Every time the tears ceased and Patty undertook to talk, just so often the floods burst forth again. Helen grew a bit impatient, and wanted to know what it was all about, but Nan gave her a warning glance, that curbed her curiosity.

For Nan knew Patty's temperament, and knew, too, that only some really great matter lay at the bottom of this outbreak.

At last, a point was reached, where it seemed that the tears were really exhausted, and, weak and white, Patty looked with loving gratitude into Nan's comforting eyes.

"Bless you, dear," Nan said, kissing the flushed cheek,—"here's a dry pillow, now, rest. I'm going to get you a glass of milk and a biscuit."

When Nan returned, Patty was quiet, and very sad-looking. Helen was trying to cheer her up by talking nonsense, but Patty paid little heed to her chatter.

Mechanically she took the milk that Nan brought, and nibbled at a biscuit.

"It's this, people," she said, at length, "you might as well know, first as last. Billee has thrown me over."

Helen stared, aghast, but Nan laughed.

"Oh, Patty!" she cried, "all that fuss for a simple little lovers' quarrel! Well I suppose you are a simple little lover, and I daresay Bill has no notion of it all. *What's* your fancied grievance? And, I must admit I'm relieved! I feared it was something serious."

"And it is!" flashed Patty; "I guess you'll think so when you know. I sent him a val— valentine——"

"And that upset the apple-cart? Why, why; was it a 'comic'?"

"Don't tease, Nan, it's fearful. You saw the valentine, didn't you, Bumble?"

"Yes, but I don't remember anything about it. What was it?"

"Here it is!" and Patty drew from beneath a pillow a moist, bedraggled paper, that had once been a gay, crisp sheet.

Nan took it and smoothed it out. She saw a blurred picture of two rustic lovers and with some difficulty she read the absurd lines beneath.

> " Our love is high as Heaven
> And wide as rolling sea——"

she read aloud, " that's all right, seems to me, —Little Billee can't have thrown you over for *that* sentiment! Now, I'll read further:

> The vows cannot be riven
> That bind my love and me.

[175]

Patty-Bride

Orthodox, I'm sure. Not a perfect rhyme,
perhaps, but that's not enough to quarrel over!
Let's see what comes next:

> But should our pledge be broken
>   Or should your love be dead,
> Send back this tender token
>   And let us never wed.

Why, Patty Fairfield, do you mean to say you
sent this ridiculous thing to your Little Billee!
I don't wonder he sent it back! It's silly beyond words! Why did you send such a
horror?"

"I dunno," said Patty, a little shame-facedly,
"mostly because Lieutenant Herron dared me
to, and I never will be dared. But, oh, Nan,
I don't care if it is a foolish valentine, he *did*
send it back,—and, don't you see, it says,
'Send back this tender token, and let us never
wed,'—and he *did* send it back!"

Patty's eyes were large and scared-looking,
and, though she didn't cry now, she looked as
if she were about ready to.

"But——" Nan looked bewildered,—"I
don't understand——"

"I do!" cried Helen, "and it's awful! I
don't wonder you're upset, Patty! But, hold

on, maybe somebody else got it and sent it back."

"No," and Patty forlornly showed the envelope. "See, it's his writing, mailed in Washington, yesterday—oh,—how could he? Why should he?"

"Patty Fairfield, behave yourself!" Nan gave her a little shake; "do you mean to tell me Bill Farnsworth means he returns your valentine—your love-token!"

"There it is! That's the one I sent him, and it *says* to return it if his love is dead—and, he's returned it! And that horrid Herron told me about a—a b-black-eyed b-beauty——"

"Nonsense, Patty! be sensible! It can't be——"

"Very well, how *do* you explain it? Why should I send that thing to him a few days ago, and get it back today? Why would he return it—there's no mistaking his writing, look at it—unless he meant me to take it as it's printed there! He has been bewitched by that b-black-eyed——"

"Hush, Patty! Don't talk such absolute rubbish! I know Bill Farnsworth, and I know——"

"You don't know the girl——"

" Jealous! Fie, Patty, for shame! "

" But, Nan," interposed Bumble, " as Patty says, what does it mean? I wouldn't doubt Little Billee's faith and loyalty either, only, in the face of this thing, what can we think? "

" I'll never believe Bill meant that! He's teasing you——"

" A pretty way to tease! " Patty was angry now. " And you know he isn't a tease. He never plays jokes like Kit Cameron, or Chick Channing might. No, Nan, he has been bowled over by a Washington girl and he wants to get rid of me! "

" Patty," and Nan spoke very seriously, " it isn't right for you so to doubt the man you've promised to marry. I can't, I won't believe that he means this as you take it! "

" How else can he mean it? If you'll give me a rational explanation of what he *does* mean, I'll be only too glad. I've thought and thought, and I can't imagine any meaning but the actual fact that the printed words say to send the valentine back if his love is dead,— and he did send it back! Now, for your explanation! "

" I don't know, Patty. I confess I don't. It isn't like him to do it to tease you."

" Of course, it isn't! He'd never do such a cruel, heartless thing as that,—if he still loved me. So, he *has* done the cruel thing,—and it's because he *doesn't* love me! "

" What are you going to do? " asked Helen, breaking a long silence.

" There's nothing to do," replied Patty, hopelessly. " I can't write and beg him to take me back. I have some pride! Nor can I ask what I've done to forfeit his regard. For I know I haven't done anything."

" You've flirted with Phil Van Reypen," said Helen, accusingly.

" I haven't! " flared Patty. " On the contrary, I've been very careful not to! He's flirted with me, if you like, but I've not encouraged him. You know I haven't, Nan."

" Not intentionally, dear, but you have been with him a great deal of late,—and Little Billee is of a jealous nature."

" No, it isn't that," and Patty sighed, forlornly; " I only wish it were! Then I could ask his pardon and make up and all that. No, my Billee has found somebody he likes better'n me. I'm Leah, the Forsaken,—after all! "

" Leah, nothing! " exclaimed Helen. " Patty,

if you can't cut out a little black-eyed beauty, you're no good! Don't submit so tamely! Go to Washington,—hunt up the horrid little thing, and see what she's like! Then, I'll back your beauty against her, any day!"

"Oh, hush up, Bumble! Do you suppose I'd stoop to get back a man who has thrown me over! You must be crazy! I love Bill Farnsworth,—I adore him, and I can never love anybody else; but I'll never raise a finger to whistle him back! I'm not that sort of a girl! I shall never write him again, or refer to this miserable business in any way. I'm glad Mr. Herron gave me the hint, or I might have made a fool of myself; now, I won't!"

Nan was re-reading the unlucky missive.

"It's very strange," was her comment. "I can't understand it. There is no mistaking his handwriting; there's no mistaking the words of that silly verse! But I don't like it, Patty. I'm surprised at Bill. If he had ceased to love you, why not tell you so, like a gentleman? You know, I always said——"

"Stop, Nan!" and Patty's voice was tense, while red spots burned on her cheeks, "don't you dare cast any reflection on him! My Billee is all right! He *is* a gentleman! I laid myself open to this treatment and I deserved all I've got. It was bad taste to say the least, for me to send that thing! I never should have done it, but to get more money for the committee. I was thoughtless, careless, and foolishly unwilling to let Mr. Herron think I didn't dare send it. He said ' you don't dare take the chance!' meaning that I might get back—just what I did get back! But I was so *sure* of Bill's love, so confident of his faith and loyalty, that I never dreamed there was a chance of Mr. Herron's being right!"

" He isn't right!" cried Helen. " I believe there's a mistake somewhere!"

" Just where?" asked Patty, listlessly. " If you can invent or imagine something that would explain his returning that horrid old thing, tell me! I'll be glad to know it!"

But Helen couldn't think of any plausible or even possible explanation or excuse for the return of the valentine.

For Farnsworth was *not* a practical joker, and indeed, few lovers could have been capable of such a jest as that!

The case seemed to be at a deadlock. It was incredible that Little Billee should have sent back the valentine, yet, there it was! And in-

[181]

dubitably from him. There was no possibility that any one else had written Patty's address on the big envelope. Bill's large, well-formed chirography was characteristic and unmistakable.

"There's another thing," confessed Patty, "Bill thinks I opened a letter that he sent me, sealed. And I didn't. Maybe that made him stop loving me."

The flower-face was so pathetic in its tragic grief, that Nan waxed wroth again.

"Patty," she said, "if Bill Farnsworth has really tossed you off like a discarded glove, I think Fred Fairfield will reckon with him! It's outrageous,—that's what it is!"

"Oh, no, Nan; don't let Father do anything sensational! I don't want a man who doesn't · want me! I assure you I don't! I'm no meek Griselda——"

"She was the patient one," put in Helen.

"Well, I'm not patient, either! I'm—oh, I'm just miserable! I wish you would both clear out, and let me alone!"

"Well, we won't," said Nan, determinedly. "But, I'll tell you what we are going to do. You dress yourself all up and we'll all go down town and lunch at the gayest and giddiest place

we can find, and then we'll go to a foolish
matinée,—the most hilarious one there is on the
boards,—and then, we'll get a new start, and
when we come home we can talk this over with
your father, and see what's what in the Fairfield household!"

Patty demurred, saying she didn't want to go,
but Nan was inexorable, and at last Patty
yielded. But only on the condition that they
would give her half an hour alone first, to
think things out.

This was granted, and Patty was left alone
and undisturbed for the stipulated time.

When Nan came again to the room, she found
Patty not yet dressing, but looking far more
cheerful.

" I've thought it out," she greeted Nan; " and
here's the result. I'm going to keep faith in my
Little Billee, until he tells me with his own lips
that he's tired of me, and loves another girl.
I can't see any way to hope this isn't so, but
I'm going to keep my faith, till I know more,
—anyway. Because, Nan," her voice fell to a
whisper, "if I don't, I'll go crazy! When I
remember all he has said to me,—all his faith
in me, all his protestations of undying, unfail-
ing love, I can't *believe* it's all swept away by

some new face! Think how long Bill has cared
for me———"

"That's right, Patty, look at it like that. It's
a whole lot better."

As a matter of fact, Nan, too, had thought it
over very seriously, and she could see no explanation but Bill Farnsworth's deep perfidy.
She could conceive of no theory that would fit
the facts, save the hint that Herron had
dropped, that Bill had been enslaved by a
sparkling little brunette, full of the Southern
charm and fascination.

It was not like Farnsworth, but Nan realised
that men are not always masters of their
fates.

She carried out her plan, and took the two
girls to luncheon and then to the theatre, and
she was glad to see that Patty's poise had returned to her, and though not exactly cheerful,
she was at least, calm and composed.

Whether this was due to the gay entertainment, or to her avowed faith in her recreant
lover, Nan didn't know. But she was glad that
Patty was outwardly pleasant and placid, whatever might be the turmoil in her heart.

They returned home about six o'clock, and
as they entered, Jane, the housemaid, told Patty

there had been a long-distance telephone call for her, during the afternoon.

"And whoever it was," Jane said, "promised to call you again later,—at half-past six."

"All right," said Patty, her heart bounding with hope that the call might be from Washington. But it was improbable, for owing to the difficulties and delays in getting a good connection, Bill rarely could take time for this method of communication.

Still outwardly serene, she went to her room and took off her wraps, and then returned to the library to await the expected call.

"Of course, it will be Bill," said Helen, comfortingly.

"Of course it won't," Patty returned, drearily, and then she waited.

CHAPTER XII

LENA AND BILL

TO get the right view of certain matters, let us go back a few days, and transport ourselves to Washington.

On the thirteenth of February, Captain Farnsworth was busily engaged at his desk work, when Lena Richards came flying in at his doorway.

"Don't scold!" she cried, by way of forestalling his objections to her presence; "I *must* talk to somebody, and it might as well be *you!*"

"It might as well be the President of the United States, and all his Cabinet, as far as I'm concerned," and Farnsworth scowled at her, "but I'd rather you'd choose anybody than my unworthy self! What shall I do with you, Lena? You're a little nuisance! Must I lock and bar the door to keep you out?"

"Now, now, don't be cross to a poor little lonesome girlie, what hasn't got anybody to consult. Lemme ask you a few questions, do!"

Lena and Bill

Lena was a wheedlesome creature, and quite in the habit of having her own way. She laughed at Bill's frown and as she plumped herself down in an armchair, she spread out on Farnsworth's desk a number of gay valentines.

"This," she began, "is for Dick Selden. Isn't it a dandy! And this one is for my own Daddy. Won't he be surprised to get one?"

Lena chuckled happily, and looked up into Bill's face for a show of approval.

She seemed only a child; her sixteen years sat lightly on her slim little shoulders, and her dark, winsome face was lighted with such a glow of happy anticipation, that good-natured Farnsworth couldn't bear to speak shortly to her.

"All right, Baby," he said, good-humouredly, "show me your valentines, and get it over with. Which one is for me?"

"Oh, that I haven't here! Of course I wouldn't show you that one!" A merry laugh rippled from the rosy lips. "And you'll send me one, won't you, Captain?"

"Why, I hadn't thought of doing so. In fact, I hadn't thought of sending any."

"What! Not to your sweetheart? Not to

that lovely angel-faced girl whose pictures are all about here? I'm ashamed of you! What *will* she think?"

Farnsworth suddenly realised his defection. "But," he said, "she'll forgive me. Patty will understand. She knows I'm terribly busy—more than busy,—I'm all in a moil, and working night and day to straighten it out——"

"But, Captain! That isn't enough to excuse not sending a valentine to the girl of your heart! Whee! If I were engaged to a man, and if he didn't send me a valentine! I'd break that engagement so quick he wouldn't know what hit him! Fie, fie, Captain! You're a peach of a lover, you are!"

Lena had risen and was dancing about the room. A restless elf, she rarely sat still long, and loved to fly about, looking at things here and there, poking and prying curiously into books or papers, and really bothering the life out of Farnsworth. Many times he had concluded to move to other quarters, where he might be free from her interruptions, but this house suited him so well otherwise, and, too, he was so busy, he disliked to take the necessary time to make the change.

But Lena's accusation gave his big, true heart

a thrill. Was he really negligent of Patty? His own Posy-face Patty,—whom he loved with all his great soul! He knew he was not a society man, not much of an observer of the lighter conventions, and he wondered if Patty would expect a valentine from him, and be disappointed at not receiving it.

"I'll send her some flowers," he exclaimed; "I can telegraph a florist in New York and have them delivered tomorrow,—that's the day, isn't it, Lena?"

"Yes; but flowers are so—so impersonal, and careless. You ought to send her a real valentine. Here, you can have one of these."

"Can I? Really! Oh, you dear little girl! That would help a lot,—for I haven't time to go out to the shops. Let me take your prettiest one, and I'll pay you what it cost, and you can buy another."

"All right," and Lena nodded her pretty head. "That goes! Now, I've only one here that I want to spare. This one."

Lena held up a pretty looking affair. It had a picture of an affectionate pair, leaning over a rustic stile, and surrounded by hearts and darts and Cupids and rose garlands.

The lines printed inside the leaf, were:

[189]

Patty-Bride

" Our love is high as Heaven
    And wide as rolling sea:
The vows cannot be riven
    That bind my love and me.
But should our pledge be broken
    Or should your love be dead,
Send back this tender token
    And let us never wed."

Farnsworth looked at it carelessly. "All right," he said, " if that's the only one available, I'll have to take that one. It's all right, isn't it?"

"Yes, it's a beauty! It cost a dollar,—but it's good work."

"Cheap at the price!" laughed Farnsworth, taking out his pocketbook. "I don't care such a lot for the sentiment, however. The first part is all right, but that second stanza is ridiculous!"

"How, ridiculous? I think it's lovely! You don't think she'll send it back, do you?"

"I do not! Our vows cannot be riven,—as your poet hath it. But I could have made up a better jingle myself! That's what I ought to have done! Made a real valentine for my sweetheart! Oh, I wish I weren't so over-

worked! Well, some day I'll make up to her
for this enforced neglect. Now, be off, Lena,
if you don't, I'll pitch you out,—neck and
crop!"

"Oh, all right, Captain; but I was going to
say if you'd address your valentine, I'd post it
along with mine. There's none too much time,
you know."

"Thank you, Lena, you're a good little thing.
And I'm a bear,—a cross one, sometimes, I
fear. Will you forgive me, and take my valentine with yours?"

"'Course I will. Write the directions."

So Farnsworth dashed off Patty's name and
address on the big envelope, and Lena ran away
with it.

So, you see!

Of course, the valentine Bill sent Patty was
the counterpart of the one she sent him, and
when you know all, you'll find out that this
wasn't such a strange coincidence as it might
seem.

And of course, the valentine that Patty received, and that caused her such paroxysms of
woe, was the one Lena mailed and *not* the
return of the one she had sent to Farnsworth.

It was a fine mixup, and Cupid, the little god

of Love, must have flown madly about in his dismay and despair of ever getting it straightened out.

Now, as is well known, the extra mail occasioned by the observance of the festival of St. Valentine, often causes delays in transmission. Which explains why both these important missives we're interested in, reached their respective destinations a couple of days after they were normally due.

And Patty, as we have seen, was pretty well broken up over the receipt of hers! Naturally, she supposed it to be the one she sent, returned to her by Farnsworth, and no one could wonder that she did think this.

And so, when Captain Farnsworth found in his mail a big square envelope addressed in Patty's well-known, well-loved handwriting, he knew it for a valentine before he opened it.

"Bless her heart!" he said to himself. "Dear little girl to send me a valentine! And I'm jolly glad I sent her one! I must thank that bothersome little Lena for that!"

He opened the envelope, and to his astonishment, he drew out what seemed to be the very valentine he had sent Patty.

Lena and Bill

"What!" he cried aloud, a puzzled frown coming over his face.

He looked at it carefully; being exactly the same, he naturally thought Patty had returned his missive.

Bewildered, he read the lines, which he had scarcely sensed as he hastily glanced them over before sending.

> "Send back this tender token
> And let us never wed."

Patty had sent it! Had returned his "tender token!"

"Should your love be dead"—was he, then, to infer that Patty's love was dead? His Patty! Never, in a million years! If ever a girl was true blue, that girl was Patty Fairfield, —his own Patty Blossom! There could be no two opinions about that!

With a sudden jerk, he picked up the telephone and called for New York.

It took a long time to get the connection, and Captain Farnsworth grew more and more impatient. He did not storm at the operator, that was not his way. He patiently waited "just a minute," till scores of minutes flew by, and at last he heard Jane's voice.

Patty-Bride

No, Miss Patty was not at home; she would be home about six. He would call up again? Very well. Good-bye.

Farnsworth strode up and down his room. It was only half-past three, he would call her about half-past six. Meantime—he must work. But the big man couldn't settle himself to work. The thing was so inexplicable, so disturbing. Had Patty meant it for a joke? Had she meant to tease him? If so it was a bit of bad taste,—and Patty was never guilty of bad taste. He couldn't understand it at all.

He tried to make out his reports, and of course, he succeeded in doing so, but it was a process greatly interrupted by long periods of distracted thought.

Suppose Patty really meant it! Bosh! Meant it! His Patty? Never! He would believe anything but that! Could it have been a mistake? Did she slip his valentine in an envelope which she had addressed to him for the purpose of sending another one,—and then she had mixed them up?

No; Patty was never careless, and least of all, where he was concerned. She was efficient, always, and he had had too much correspondence with her not to know how careful she was. And then, came to his mind dark thoughts of Philip Van Reypen.

Suppose,—just *suppose,* Patty had found that she preferred Phil to himself,—could she have chosen a better or more definite way to tell him so?

" Should your love be dead! "

The big man writhed at the thought. He put it out of his mind as unworthy of him and unworthy of his love. And yet, that would explain it,—and what else would? What else could? But that explanation he refused to accept. Patty, his own gentle dear little Patty, he wouldn't be cruel,—but—if she had such a thing to tell him, she would choose some way that seemed to her the least cruel—he knew that!

Was she using his means—as he had unwittingly given her the chance,—oh, why *had* he sent that foolish thing? It was silly,—it was absurd,—it was bad taste on his part!

But Lena had brought it, and it had seemed to him silly, but harmless.

He worried and fretted, fumed and scowled, but he could come to no satisfactory conclusion or explanation.

[195]

Patty-Bride

He looked at his watch until he almost wore it out, only to find each time that but a moment or two had elapsed.

At last he gave up trying to work and went out for a walk.

The clear cold air freshened his brain but his heart still had a dull, queer ache in it. He did a few errands, forcing himself to concentrate his mind in their accomplishment, and at last the slow-going clock-hands crawled around to half-past six.

Back in his own rooms, Bill called New York again, and asked for Patty's number.

The connection was a good one, and he finally heard the well-beloved voice say, "Hello,— Little Billee!"

"Oh, Patty!" he cried, explosively, "oh, Patty Blossom! When will you marry me? What day? Tell me, quick!"

"Why—why—you sent back———"

"No, I didn't! I didn't send back anything! Never mind that fool valentine business! Answer my question, quick! Sometimes they snap off the connection, and if they did *that* I'd go wild! *When*, Patty?"

"Why—oh—any time! Bill, dear,—any time!"

"Bless you, darling! But what day? what date? Tell me."

"Oh,—I can't——"

"Yes, you can! Now,—and make it soon!"

"Well, say in October——"

"October your grandmother! Say April."

"Oh, nonsense, Bill, I can't! And this is no thing to decide over a telephone! You come up here——"

"I can't,—not for a few days, and I've got to know this thing now,—see? NOW!"

"Well, say June, then."

"No! you may say May, but not a day later. Say your birthday, that's in May."

"May's an unlucky month——"

"Not for us,—it won't be! On your birthday, then——"

"Wait a minute, Bill, what made you return my valentine?"

"What made you return mine?"

"I didn't!"

"*I* didn't! Oh, Patty, I see it,—it has just dawned on me! We sent duplicates! Where'd you get yours?"

"At a bazaar thing——"

"Yes, I see; and I got mine from—well,—I got it."

" Where? "

" No matter now. I bought it and paid for it; and they chanced to be just alike! Puzzle it out at your leisure. Now, Posy-face, I'm coming to New York just as soon as I can manage it, but it may be a week or so,—I hope not, I hope to get there in a couple of days, but all I can say is, I'll do the best I can, and you begin to get ready for that May affair."

" Not May, Bill—June! "

" Oh, why? *why* not May? Well, wait till I see you, and perhaps I can persuade you to say May."

" Well, we'll see, but I refuse to decide it over a telephone! Nobody *ever* did! "

" As if that mattered! Well, you get busy with your preparations, and we'll see——"

" Now, you must say good-bye, dear. You know this is long distance and not a local call! "

" I don't care if it is! Tell me something,— Patty! "

" Oh, I can't tell you *that* at long distance! "

" No; and if I hear your voice without seeing you, much longer, I'll go off my head! Good-bye, then, you darling, Patty Blossom,——"

Lena and Bill

"Oh, Little Billee! Don't! Somebody'll hear you!"

"Let 'em! Good-bye, dearest,—my Best Beloved!"

"Good-bye!"

Patty hung up the receiver, and sat very still, her eyes shining like two big blue stars.

She hadn't quite straightened out the valentine mixup in her mind yet, but she didn't care! It was all right! Little Billee loved her just the same as ever,—if not more! And she had promised to marry him in June! It was a sudden step. She had realised she was engaged to him,—and would marry him some day; but she never had, even in her own mind, set any definite date.

"Well," said Helen, coming in, "I discreetly stayed out, while you were telephoning, now I think I might be told if the call *was* from Washington."

"It was!" answered Patty; "it most certainly was!"

"And you're not crying as torrentially as you were?"

"I am not!" and Patty smiled like a Chessy cat. "In fact, I think I may assure you I shall never cry again; at least, not if I continue to feel as happy as I do at this present speaking."

"Good for you, my fairy cousin! Now,—tell old Bumble all about it!"

So Patty told her.

"Well, of all things! Do you mean that he, just by chance, sent you a valentine exactly like the one you sent him?"

"Yes; and I suppose they're all over. You know every year there's some funny or clever one that has a vogue everywhere."

"Queer, for him to select that for you!"

"It was, but I don't care! He did, and I did, so we can't blame each other. But I was the baddy one, because I distrusted him! He hadn't a doubt of me! When he,—as he supposed,—got back the one he sent me, he called up and asked me to set our wedding-day!"

"Did he, really? Oh, Patty, that's the sort of a man to marry! I always did like him, now I think he's just perfectly stunning!"

"I do, too, and I'm ashamed of my doubts and fears."

"Oh, that's all right, he'll never know."

"Yes, he will, I shall tell him. And maybe he'll be so disappointed in me, and so hurt, that——"

"That he'll break off the engagement! Oh,

yes! Oh, certainly! Patty, you are a goose, and always will be! Never let him know what a goose you are, or he sure will throw you over!"

"Oh, I guess not!" Patty smiled happily.

"Well, when is the day? What did he say?"

"I wouldn't say positively,—but, oh, Bumble, he's so impatient!"

"Of course he is! Any real lover would be, and especially any one who is expecting to marry Patty Fairfield!"

CHAPTER XIII

AN IMPORTANT DOCUMENT

PATTY was walking up and down the library, waiting for Little Billee. He had written and he had telegraphed and he had telephoned, and every message changed or contradicted the previous one, and Patty was nervous.

She flew from one chair to another, she flung herself on the davenport, and back to the window-seat; she pulled aside the curtains and stared down the street, in fact, she flew around, Bumble declared, like a hen with her head off.

" Fly, if you like, Patty," Nan said, kindly; " it may help some."

It was three o'clock, and she had expected Bill momentarily since one. And at last she saw him! The big man came swinging round a corner and looking up, saw Patty's face at the window.

He paused at the sight, and the two stood, beaming at each other.

An Important Document

"Oh, there he is!" Nan cried. "Come, Bumble, let's leave them to themselves for a few minutes."

"A few hours!" Patty called out, as the two slipped from the room, and then Farnsworth came in.

He found a Patty smiling with joy, not nervous now, but a lovely shining-eyed girl, with welcoming arms outstretched and a soft flush tinting her cheeks.

"Blossom Girl!" he cried, and then he clasped her in a big whole-souled embrace, that nearly swept her off her feet.

Close he held her, in a happy silence, then he gently lifted the flower-face and kissed the quivering lips.

"Oh, my dearest, my Best Beloved, I thought I'd never get here! The trains crawled, the waits were interminable! But I'm here, and I have you in my arms and nothing else matters!"

"You dear thing!" Patty said, timidly reaching up to caress his strong, firm chin with her little fingers, "I'd forgotten you're so—so enormous!"

Farnsworth's laugh rang out.

"There *is* a lot of me, isn't there? But I'm

all yours, so you must get used to seeing me round. Would you rather I were less enormous, Patty?"

"No, indeed! I wouldn't have you changed in any respect! You're just right! But you make me feel small!"

"And you are. My little Patty *Petite*. I'm glad, too, 'cause I like you much better this way. You see, I can pick you up and put you wherever I please."

Farnsworth picked Patty up like a child, and placed her on the big davenport, then sat down beside her.

"Now, I'm happy! Can we sit here forever, —or do we have to be ordinary citizens and chum with the family?"

"They'll let us alone a little while, and then I s'pect Nan and Bumble will come in."

"Oh, pshaw! I hoped I'd have you all to myself. Can't we send them to a matinée, or something?"

"It's too late for that. Here they come now, Little Billee! Take your arm away!"

"Shan't! They know you're mine, and I've a perfect right to have my arm round you!"

"But—it isn't done! It isn't conventional!"

An Important Document

"I make my own conventions! Hello, Bumble! How d'you do, Mrs. Fairfield? Excuse this small parcel I hold in my left arm, but I can't let go of it."

Farnsworth's bonny smile was so glad and gay that Nan smiled in sympathy.

"All right," she said, "don't mind us."

"We don't," said Patty, and she cuddled contentedly in Big Bill's outstretched arm, as they returned to the sofa.

"You see," Farnsworth explained, "I've had the dickens of a time to get away at all, and everything interfered and detained me. I can only stay a few hours,——"

"What!" cried Patty, "you're going right back? Tonight?"

"Yes, dear; I'm on a big mission,—two big missions, in fact, one connected with my country and one with my sweetheart. I try not to let them get mixed up,—but it's difficult to give undivided attention to either."

"What'd you come for," demanded Patty, "if you have to go right away again?"

"I came, my child, to make sure you will name a certain date, that will be to me, the most momentous in American history. I must get *that* settled before I go to work in earnest to

[205]

help win the war! And you said you couldn't do it over the telephone."

"This way is nicer," and Patty nestled against his shoulder.

"For bare-faced love-makers, you two are pretty outspoken," commented Bumble, smiling at them.

"'Scuse!" said Patty, without moving. "We wouldn't under ordinary conditions, but realise, please, that our love-making has to be done when we can get a chance,—which is awful seldom. If you don't want to play audience,—there is another course open to you."

"No, thank you, I *won't* run away!" and Bumble settled down to stay. "I want to hear all the plans and arrangements,—and oh, Patty, when is the day to be?"

"I'm cornered, I see, and I suppose I may as well decide now as any time. Let's say June—about the middle of June. How's that, Little Billee?"

"Next best to May, if you can't be ready for May. How about the first of June?"

"No, 'long about the middle or latter part. I've a heap to do. I can't get married without a lot of embroidered linen things——"

An Important Document

" Oh, have a shower! " cried Bumble.

" Nonsense! I don't want a shower! I mean really lovely things,—all hand-embroidered,—oh, Little Billee, shall we live in a *house?*"

" Why, I had supposed so,—but if you prefer a tree——"

" No; I mean a house or an apartment, or what? "

" Goodness, Agnes! *I* don't know. Live wherever you like,—and I'll live there too."

" In Washington? "

" That I don't know," and Farnsworth looked suddenly serious. " It all depends on the war developments, Patty. I may have to go to France."

" All right,—I'll go along."

" But perhaps you can't,—it will be on a special mission——"

Tears came to Patty's eyes. " Whatever your country calls you to do, you must do, of course," she said, slowly, " but if you go to France and leave me here—I'll go with you,—so there, now! "

" It may not come to that," Farnsworth sighed a little wearily; " and we won't cross the bridge until we come to it. You go ahead as fast as you can, embroidering your tidies and tablespreads, and——"

"Oh, I shan't embroider them. I'll have them done,—in the trousseau shops,—oh, they will be lovely!"

"You goose!" cried Bumble. "I believe you think more of your trousseau than of your husband!"

Patty made no answer to this, save a flashing glance at Farnsworth, which seemed to assure him that Bumble's notion was a mistaken one.

"Tell us about the valentines," Nan said, "however did you come to get one just like Patty's?"

"Wasn't it queer?" assented Bill. "And, if you ask me, I think they were silly, stupid things, anyway! How'd *you* come to get it, Patty?"

"On a dare," Patty laughed. "Lieutenant Herron——"

"Who's he?"

"One of my new army friends. Oh, Little Billee, I've so much to tell you, and no time to tell it in!"

"That's so! and first of all, I must ask you if you opened a sealed note before I told you you might."

An Important Document

"No; I didn't." Patty's blue eyes met Farnsworth's blue ones with a gaze of unmistakable honesty.

"I knew you didn't, of course," he said, perplexedly, "but the trouble is, who did? Somebody must have done so, to know that I thought of coming up to New York. It was important that it shouldn't be known."

"But who could have done it?"

"Where was the letter?"

"In the pocket of my fur stole: that has a most secure clasp-button, and I'm sure it wasn't meddled with."

"Patty!" cried Bumble, "you know that spy thing, who dressed up as a woman——"

"What!" exclaimed Farnsworth.

Eagerly Patty and Bumble together told the story of the missing chaperon and the masquerading pastry-cook.

Farnsworth looked very grave.

"A spy, undoubtedly," he said; "in Herron's employ."

"Oh, not Lieutenant Herron! Why, he's one of our own soldiers!"

"Forget it, Patty. And you, too, Helen. Never mention the subject to any human being. Much depends on that. I can trust you?"

"Oh, yes!" vowed both girls.

"Did I do wrong, dear?" asked Patty, anxiously.

"Not knowingly, sweetheart; but you must be very careful. I use you as my little helper, but if it is known, I must not do it. Now, Patty, here is another paper, that I want to leave in your care for a couple of days. Hide it as carefully as you can, and when I tell you to, then, mail it."

"I will," and Patty took the letter. "I'll put it in this desk, now,—see, it has a secret compartment."

Patty went to an antique mahogany desk, and in sight of them all, she secreted the important document.

"That's probably all right," and Farnsworth sighed with relief. "I was a bit fidgetty about having it in my pockets any longer. Now, don't touch that desk, or open the secret drawer until I tell you to post the packet. Somebody might see you poking about."

"But there are no spies here, Billee."

"They are everywhere. No place is surely safe from them. Don't worry, or even think about them. But just obey orders, unquestioningly, like the loyal little patriot you are!"

An Important Document

" All right; just as you say," and Patty smiled
at her commander.

" Why, look who's here! " Bumble cried, and
Fred Fairfield came in.

" Hello, Farnsworth! Well, but I'm glad to
see you! You're looking fine, barring a deep
line of care and responsibility that has fur-
rowed itself into your brow."

" Oh, I'm all right, especially now that I'm
back home."

" Home it is, my boy. You're a pretty big
order for a son, but I'm all ready to adopt
you."

" All right, Dad, give me fatherly advice
when needed."

And then to Farnsworth's deep regret, Philip
Van Reypen came to call.

The two men met courteously and were outwardly calm, but in each heart rankled a dis-
taste of the other.

Perhaps it was absurd, but Farnsworth was
jealous of Philip, and though confident of
Patty's love and loyalty, he hated to think of
Van Reypen in New York while he must be
in Washington.

As to Philip, he was frankly envious of Little
Billee, and moreover, was determined to cut

him out and regain Patty for himself if it could possibly be done. Phil was not dishonourable, —at least, he didn't think he was,—for he deemed all fair in love and war.

But Captain Farnsworth was very glad when he learned that Van Reypen must of necessity be in Wilmington almost all the time. To be sure, his leave of absence seemed to occur very often, but after all he didn't really live in New York now, and that cheered Little Billee's heart.

" When will you fly with me? " Van Reypen asked of Patty, and he purposely gave his question a sentimental flavour that startled Farnsworth by its implication.

" Not till you're an experienced airman," returned Patty, gaily, and then Bill realised what was meant.

" Patty! " he said, severely, " you are *never* to go in an aeroplane,—I forbid it! "

He spoke far more sternly, even harshly than he meant to, for the bare idea of her so risking her life appalled him, and with the added awfulness of her going up with Van Reypen, Little Billee felt indeed aghast.

" No? " said Patty, pouting a little; " oh, but I want to! "

An Important Document

"Never! Understand? It is an order!"

The positiveness of Farnsworth's commands was quite softened by the sweetness of his tone, but Patty was perverse, and she replied, "I shan't promise."

"Oh, yes, you will, dear,—you'll promise because I ask it."

Farnsworth stepped nearer to her, and with one hand raised her chin until her gaze met his. His strong, loving glance conquered, and won by the deep love she saw in his eyes, Patty said, simply, "I promise."

"That's all right," and Bill smiled at her, needing no reiteration or reassurance. Her simple word was sufficient.

Van Reypen said nothing, but he gave Patty a quizzical glance.

"Yes, indeed," she replied to his insinuation. "I love to be bossed!"

"Oh, Patty, don't lose your wilfulness,— that's one of your charms."

"Not any more. You don't know, Phil, how an engaged girl loves to be told what she may and what she may not do. And, incidentally, I've no desire to break my neck before my wedding-day!"

"Oh, don't think I'd take you flying until I was sure of my own powers."

"Powers are not all of it," Farnsworth said, "accidents are unavoidable, even in the best regulated airships. But that matter is settled. How do you like the air game, Phil?"

"Top notch! I was cut out for an aviator, —I feel it. There's no sport like it! Though I don't take it exactly as a sport. I'm making a very serious business of it."

"Good for you! That's the way to talk. Now, people and friends, I'm going to ask you all to go away from this place and let me have a little time alone with Patty, or else, stay here and let us go somewhere else."

Patty gasped at this high-handed suggestion, but was truly pleased, for she hated to have Farnsworth and Van Reypen together, and too, she wanted to see Little Billee alone.

Nan, always helpful, hustled them all out to another room, and left the lovers in possession of the library.

"He is splendid," said Bumble as they went to the family sitting-room. "Doesn't he look fine in uniform!"

"Great," agreed Van Reypen, who was not at all petty, "he's a fine old chap. And, after

yours truly, I don't know any one more worthy
of our Patty."

"You're both so splendid," said Bumble, with
a flattering glance, "I should think Patty would
feel 'how happy could I be with either, were
t'other dear charmer away.'"

"That's what I hope," declared Phil, who
made no secret of his wishes regarding Patty.

"But you're both away most of the time.
I'm going away too, tomorrow."

"Home?"

"Oh, no. To visit a friend in East Ninety-
fifth Street. She invited me for a week, but
I'm only going to stay a couple of days,—unless
I like it very much, then I might stay longer."

"Can't I take you there? When are you
going?"

"Oh, no, thank you. Nan will send me, of
course. I go tomorrow afternoon. Patty
won't miss me, she's so busy ordering linen."

"How she does love pretty things."

"Oh, she does! She's just the one to get
married, if only to get up a trousseau. Me,
when I'm married, I won't know whether I've
any worldly goods or not!"

"You never do, anyhow, do you?" said Nan,
laughing.

Meantime, Patty was discussing great and important matters with Farnsworth.

"I leave all plans and arrangements to you," he was saying; "I believe that's the bride's prerogative anyhow, but I'm really ignorant of such matters. Personally, I'd rather just be married to you, and run away from everybody,—without any bells on,—but it's as you say."

"Nay, nay, Pauline! Little Patty has to have a wedding, as is a wedding! Not an awful big crowd and not a gorgeous pageant, but a nice sweet pretty home wedding, with lots of white satin ribbons!"

"Not tied onto trunks and things!"

"Oh, no! Of course, not that! I mean aisles of it, and white stanchions——"

"What in the world are those?"

"Florists' posts to hold up the garlands that make the aisle through which your bride shall come to you!"

"Patty Blossom! When you say those things you do look so sweet! How can I wait till June?"

"Oh, the time will just fly! By the way, dear, *why* can't I go up in a flying machine? Everybody does."

[216]

An Important Document

" Yes, and the majority of them come down with broken bones."

" Oh, not the majority! "

" Well, a large minority, then. But, that matter is settled, dearest, once for all. You're not to do it, see? "

" Why? "

" Because I forbid it. Is that enough? "

" No; that isn't quite enough! Here's the real reason why! " Patty smiled and whispered, " Because I love you! "

" Patty Precious! How happy you make me when you're sweet and docile like that. Of course you know it's my love for you that makes me forbid your risking your life."

" I know it. Little Billee, wasn't it funny about those valentines? "

" Indeed it was. What did you mean by a dare? "

" Just that! Lieutenant Herron said I wouldn't dare send it to you, lest you send it back! And I knew you wouldn't, and so I dared! And then——"

" And then you thought I did! Oh, you *dear* little goose! "

" I couldn't help thinking so at first. How did you happen to get the one you sent? "

"Why, little Lena,—the youngster where I live,——"

"Oh, is she a little black-haired beauty?"

"A little black-haired witch! Yes, she's a good-looking kiddy——"

"How old?"

"Sixteen, I believe. What, jealous!"

"N-no; but you don't like her much, do you?"

"She's a little nuisance! I'd fly the coop, only I'm well fixed there and it's a bother to move."

"Did she tell you to send it to me?"

"No, not exactly. She said I ought to send you a valentine, and, honestly, Patty, I own up I hadn't thought of it! So, as she had some extra ones I took one and paid her for it. That's all."

"Sort of funny,—and funny they should be alike. You see, Mr. Herron practically forced me to send mine, and this little girl made you send yours!"

"Well, there's no harm done, is there? It didn't bother me when I received what might seem to be a ' returned token.' For I trust you, Patty, my Blessing, and nothing could ever make you believe you false or fickle unless you told me so yourself. So never fear what they call 'misunderstandings' for I shall come straight to you and make you understand! That's the meaning, to my mind, of our faith and trust."

"My dear big Little Billee! That's the meaning to my mind, too. And to my heart. My whole love is yours——"

"Till death do us part," Farnsworth added, reverently.

CHAPTER XIV

HELEN'S ADVENTURE

"OH, Nan, *do* let me have my own way for once!"

Bumble's flashing brown eyes looked troubled, but determined.

"I know my way perfectly," she went on. "The car can leave me at the concert and then take you on to your meeting. Then after the concert, I can hop into a taxicab and go right up to Millicent's without a bit of trouble!"

"You could, of course, Helen, if you were like other people. But you're so rattle-pated, you'd just as likely go down town as up,—and find yourself at the Battery."

"No, I won't, Nan, honest, I won't. I've only to tell the driver 783 East Ninety-fifth Street, and he'll take me right there."

"You'll forget the number."

"I'll write it on. a card, and keep it in my bag. I'm not an infant, you know."

"Well, all right, dear, if you think you won't

get lost. Telephone me as soon as you're safely at your friend's, won't you?"

"Yes, I will. What time will you get home, yourself?"

"About six. But you see, Patty wants the car at five——"

"Oh, I know,—I know all about it, and that's why I insist on carrying out my own plans."

"You've sent your suitcase, haven't you?"

"Yes, that was part of my well-laid plan. You must admit, Nan, I've looked out for everything."

"Yes, you have, Helen; and I consent, for I can't see any way out of it. You see Patty is on the reception committee, and she must——"

But Helen had flown off to get ready, so Nan turned to her own affairs.

"Good-bye, Patsy Poppet," Bumble cried, a little later, as in coat and furs she looked in at Patty's door.

"How sweet you look, angel child. Who sent you the violets——"

"Philip."

"He did! And none to me?"

"He said you had ordered him not to."

"So I have; oh, me, I can't have flowers from admiring swains any more, at all, at all!"

"Don't pretend you're sorry, for I know better. You haven't an idea in your head that isn't simply and solely about Bill Farnsworth!"

"Dear, dear! As bad as that?" Patty smiled a little absently, as she went on writing a letter.

"Yes, and you're writing to him now,—I know by the lovesick way you hold your head on one side! And, moreover, my young friend, if you don't get dressed pretty soon, you'll be late for your party. It's 'most four o'clock."

"Good gracious, Bumble! I thought your concert began at three."

"It does,—but was I ever at the beginning of anything?"

Helen calmly accepted her own chronic tardiness as a foregone conclusion, and with a waved farewell, she trotted off.

She was going to her friend's house for the night, but she greatly desired to go to a concert first, and owing to the different engagements of Patty and Nan, it was inconvenient for the Fairfield car to call for her after the performance.

But she was more than willing to go to her friend's in a cab by herself, and she had the address safely tucked away in her purse.

Helen's Adventure

The concert was enthralling to Helen's music-loving soul, and she deeply regretted that her late coming had lost her so much enjoyment.

When it was over, she drifted slowly out with the rest of the crowding audience, and reached the curb, still quivering with the exaltation that fine music always aroused in her.

In a sort of absent-minded way, she suddenly realised that it was snowing hard,—very hard, indeed. A young but vigorous blizzard had set in, and though shielded by the marquise, Helen found herself well covered with snowflakes.

She stepped up to the liveried man at the curb and said:

" Will you please call a taxi for me? "

The man looked at her.

" You'll have to wait your turn, Miss, there's twelve ahead of you. This here unexpected snowstorm makes cabs in great demand."

Helen saw that many others were more or less patiently waiting and resigned herself to wait, too.

Her mind turned back to the music, and she drew out her programme to regret anew the numbers she had missed.

A long time she stood there, studying the names of the performers and their selections, —so absorbed that she did not notice the deepening dusk, the thickening snowflakes and the rapidly rising wind.

"It's fierce, Miss," the starter said to her, at last. "I'm going to get you that cab the very minute I can,—but I dunno when 'twill be."

"What?" said Bumble, looking up. "Oh, yes,—I do want a cab. Why, how it is snowing! Get one quick, please."

"I say I can't," and the man looked honestly anxious, for Helen had an irresponsible air and the hour was growing late.

"Can't you telephone for your own car, Miss," he said, by way of a hint.

"No; I can't, Patty wants it,—I mean," she suddenly realised where she was. "I mean, the others of the family need our car. I must have a cab."

"Yes, Miss, I'll do my best."

"There ain't no use," the man told her a few minutes later. "I mean there ain't no telling when I can get you a taxi; but here's a hansom cab, don't you think now, you'd better take this?"

"What? A hansom? Oh, I never do."

Helen's Adventure

"I know, Ma'am, but it's a chance, and you might have to wait a lot longer——"

"Oh, all right, perhaps it would be the best thing to do."

"And you're lucky to get me," observed the driver from his high perch, "there ain't many vacant cabs tonight."

The starter put Helen into the little vehicle, tucked the robe about her, and closed the doors, with a feeling of relief at seeing the young lady *en route* for home. Then, before he had the glass lowered he asked for the address.

"Oh, yes," and Helen opened her bag. "Wait a minute."

But a hasty and fluttering search failed to produce the written paper.

"I had it," she murmured; "I must have jerked it out with my programme. Won't you look around on the pavement, please?"

The man obligingly looked, but the snow had fallen so thickly, that there was no sign of the lost paper.

"Never mind," Helen said, "I know the number. It's 783 West Ninety-fifth Street. I remember, because it's the same number as some one's house in Philadelphia."

"You're sure, Miss?"

"Yes, I'm sure. And it's on the third floor. My friend told me so."

"All right," and the glass slid down, and the hansom started uptown.

The progress was slow, for the street traffic was enormous at that hour and greatly impeded by the storm beside.

At last they turned into Central Park, and Helen, looking out, thought that now their gait would be a little faster.

But it was decidedly slower, and after a few moments the driver opened the little trap in the roof, and called down.

"Can't make the Park, Ma'am,—too slippery."

"What?" asked Helen, not at all comprehending.

"I say, the horse can't go through the Park. The ice under the snow is too treacherous,— he'll fall down."

"What are you going to do, then?"

"Gotter go back out again, and get over to Broadway."

"Very well, do that."

It was all Greek to Helen, for she had no idea of the position of the New York streets, and it was now so dark that the lights glimmering through the storm only made a more bewildering outlook than ever.

She had no idea where she was, or where she was going, but her optimistic nature felt no fear, only annoyance at the elements.

Faster fell the snow, and slower went the horse. He stumbled frequently, and almost fell several times.

At last he did fall, and Helen was pitched forward against the glass.

Luckily, it did not break, and as she crouched in a heap, the driver reassured her from above.

"Sit tight, Miss! We'll get him up. Don't open the doors!"

Helen was thoroughly scared now, but her good sense told her that to obey the driver's advice was the best thing she could do.

And sure enough, after a time, with the help of policemen and others, the horse was somehow again on his feet and apparently uninjured.

"Now we're off," the cheery driver called down. "It's a terrible storm, but I can get you there, if we go slowly."

"Go slowly, then," Helen answered, greatly reassured by his honest, kindly accents, "but do get there!"

So they went on, now merely crawling, as the poor horse cautiously picked his steps, and now stopping altogether, as the traffic forced them to.

Helen's watch had stopped, because she had forgotten to wind it. They passed few pedestal clocks, and those she could not see for the whirling flakes. She wanted to ask the driver how late it was getting, but couldn't make him hear.

So they kept on, and at last the cab drew up to a curb and the driver got down.

"Well, Miss," he said, "you was lucky to have me,—you sure was! For, I see you was young and didn't know New York at all hardly. And I'm mighty glad to get you here without any broken bones,—I am that!"

Helen appreciated his solicitude for her welfare, and though she well knew it was, in part, a hint for a goodly fee above his regular fare, she felt that he deserved it.

She paid him generously, and bade him good night with courteous thanks.

"You all right, now?" he asked, as he looked at the brightly-lighted entrance of the apartment house.

"Oh, yes," said Helen, glancing at the number

to be sure it was 783. "This is Ninety-fifth Street, isn't it?"

"Yes, Ma'am,—good night."

"Good night and thank you."

The hansom drove away through the storm and as Helen approached the house, the door was swung open by a liveried doorman.

She went in, smiling with gladness to be once more indoors amid light and warm surroundings, and going at once to the elevator, she said, "Third floor, please."

To the maid who answered her ring at the door of the apartment, she nodded pleasantly, and said: "I'm Miss Barlow."

Then she looked around for her friend, Millicent Wheeler.

But she saw no sign of her, and instead, a strange lady came from one of the rooms, and stared at Helen.

"What is it?" she said, politely but coldly.

"I am Miss Barlow," repeated Helen, "to see Mrs. Wheeler."

"Mrs. Wheeler? There is no such person in this house."

"What! Isn't this 783, Ninety-fifth?"

"Yes; are you looking for some friend?" The voice was kinder now, for Helen's was an appealing personality, and she was evidently in a quandary, but still the strange hostess did not invite her guest to sit down.

"Yes; oh, what can be the trouble? I'm to visit Mrs. Charles Wheeler, and her address is this house,—but I'm sure she said third floor."

"There's no Mrs. Wheeler in this house at all, that I know of. You must have the wrong number."

"No; I'm sure of the number."

"May I ask your name?"

"I'm Helen Barlow, and I live in Philadelphia. I'm visiting friends in the city, and I'm to spend tonight with another friend. Oh, what *shall* I do?"

"I don't see what you can do, but stay here till morning. It's nearly eight o'clock now, and I can't send any one out in a storm like this!"

"Nearly eight! Oh, Nan will be crazy! She *said* I'd get lost!"

The lady smiled. She was beginning to believe Helen's story, though at first she had felt wary.

"I am Mrs. Lummis," she said. "I live here and have lived here a long time. I'm sorry for you, and I'll keep you over night. I won't say, with pleasure, for as a matter of fact it will put me out considerably. But I've a little too much humanity to turn you out in this storm."

Helen overlooked the coldness of the courtesy, in her relief at having found a safe, if not very hospitable shelter.

" I'm terribly sorry," she said; " I hate to put anybody out——"

" It seems to be a question between putting me out,—or, putting you out!" laughed Mrs. Lummis, " and I think it might as well be me. Come into my little drawing-room."

Helen followed her into a small but prettily furnished room and Mrs. Lummis helped her take off her wraps.

" Now wait a minute, and we'll ferret out the mystery."

The hostess took a telephone book from a stand. " What's the name of the friend you're after?"

" Mrs. Wheeler, but she has a private wire. You can't get her number. I had it but I lost it, and Central positively refused to tell it to me."

Again Mrs. Lummis looked a bit suspicious. Then, with a whole-souled burst of enthusiasm,

she said, "I don't care if your story is fishy,—
I believe in you, and I won't ask you any more
questions."

"Oh, you think I'm an impostor!" Helen
exclaimed, the fact just dawning on her. "Oh,
how *funny!*"

Her laugh was so honest and so infectious that
Mrs. Lummis laughed too, and the two became
instant friends.

"But I hate to intrude worse than ever, now,"
declared Helen.

"Oh, never mind. It can't be helped. You
can have my room, and I'll bunk on the davenport. I live alone, and—and I expected a few
friends this evening——"

"Oh, I see. But I'm no spoilsport. Just
tuck me into bed—oh, I wonder if I couldn't
go home——" She ran to the window and
looked out. "No; it's a regular blizzard!
And I *must* call up Nan! She'll be frantic!"

"Who's this Nan?"

Mrs. Lummis was a bit blunt, but she was
kindly now, and Helen replied, "Oh, that's
where I'm staying. Mrs. Fairfield. I know
her number, may I call her?"

"You'll scare the wits out of her, if you tell

her you're in some strange house. But,—would she send for you?"

"I don't know. It's such a storm! She'd probably say if I'm safe under cover to stay here."

"Well, tell her then."

"But I know she'll worry. She told me, you see, I'd get lost,—and I did. I don't see how it happened!"

"I do. You got the wrong house. That's certain. Maybe the wrong number or street—oh, say, didn't you want *East* Ninety-fifth?"

"Why I don't know! Maybe I did! I always forget that East or West matters!"

"Oh, you little goose! *Why* did they let you out alone?"

"They said I oughtn't to come alone,—but I begged so hard."

"Well, that's it. You wanted East and you got West."

"Can't I go over East now?"

"Gracious, no! It's across the Park!"

"No; I can't cross the Park. The horse tried, and had to come out."

"Well, I see it all, now. And I'll take care of you. Do you want to tell your Fairfield friends?"

Helen considered. "I think I'll tell them that I'm all right," she said at last. "I mean, I won't tell them what really has happened,— but let them think for tonight that I'm at Mrs. Wheeler's."

Again that look of suspicion crossed Mrs. Lummis' face.

"Now stop!" Helen laughed. "I'm only doing it to save them anxiety. Mrs. Fairfield will worry all night, and my cousin will nearly go crazy."

"Well, do as you like. Then I'll give you some supper and put you to bed, for I'm telling you frankly, I'm *not* asking you to spend the evening with me."

She bustled away and Helen called up Nan.

"For goodness sake, Bumble, why didn't you call sooner? I've feared all sorts of things!"

"Nonsense, it's all right, Nan. I called you as soon as I could get around to it. Good night, now, I'm in a hurry. Bye-bye!"

Helen hung up the receiver, knowing that Nan couldn't call her back. Then, with her usual acceptance of circumstances she shook off all worry, and sat down to the pleasant little supper Mrs. Lummis offered her.

And not long after, knowing that her hostess

so wished it, Helen suggested that she should retire.

"I'm giving you my room," said Mrs. Lummis, " and I hope you'll sleep well. You must be pretty much exhausted."

"I'm not," returned Helen, "I think it's a lark! But don't fear, I won't intrude. Give me a magazine or book to read, and I'll disappear till morning. Lock me in, if you like."

"Oh, no," and the lady laughed; "I'm not afraid of your appearing at my party. Good night, my dear."

CHAPTER XV

A DESPERATE SITUATION

L EFT to herself, Bumble thought over the situation and laughed. As usual, she had got into a scrape, and, also as usual, she had fared very luckily.

Suppose instead of the kind Mrs. Lummis, she had found a disagreeable hostess! But she had fallen on her feet, and with her care-free nature she bothered herself not a whit about unpleasant possibilities.

She wandered about the pretty little bedroom, feeling very grateful for the safe harbour from the stormy night. She read a little, and then sat at the well-furnished toilet table to take down her hair.

She could hear guests arriving, and though of no mind to eavesdrop, she could not help overhearing their light talk and chatter.

Helen was not curious by nature, and paid no attention to the voices until the name of Lieutenant Herron was mentioned.

A Desperate Situation

But then the voices were lowered, and she caught no connected sentences.

A little ashamed of herself for listening at all to talk not meant for her ears, Bumble went to bed and was soon sound asleep.

Next morning Mrs. Lummis tapped at the door, and entered cheerily.

" Sleep well, little girl? Yes? That's good. Now for a bath and some breakfast, then I'm going to pack you off. Sorry to speed my parting guest so hastily, but I have to go out of town on an early train."

Helen sprang out of bed, truly sorry to inconvenience her kind benefactor.

She made especial haste with her dressing and soon the two were seated at a cosy breakfast.

Mrs. Lummis asked a good many questions and out of the kindness of her heart Helen replied in full. Suddenly she realised that she was divulging secrets. Without thinking, she had told the story of the day at the Country Club and the masquerading man, who, they suspected, had surreptitiously opened the letter that was in the pocket of Patty's fur stole.

Mrs. Lummis was greatly interested, and urged further details, and it was not until Bumble had told of Bill's sometimes giving

Patty important letters to hide, that she bethought herself of her indiscretion.

She had even told of the secret drawer in the old desk, where Patty concealed the papers, and the realisation of her mistake almost stunned her.

"Don't tell, will you?" she pleaded. "I oughtn't to have told that!"

Of a sudden Mrs. Lummis' eyes gleamed brightly.

"It's all right," she said, a trifle absent-mindedly, and rising abruptly she went to the telephone.

She called a number and presently Helen heard her talking in a foreign language.

Helen could understand no word, but she was quick-witted and it seemed to her that Mrs. Lummis was divulging important information to some one exceedingly interested.

At last she caught what was, she felt sure, the house number of the Fairfield home.

Frightened and appalled, she sat wondering what she must do.

She had heard more or less spy talk, but she knew nothing of such matters definitely. However she felt she must warn Patty, and tell her what she had inadvertently done. The horror

A Desperate Situation

and regret of her deed was almost swallowed up in the necessity for immediate action.

Helen was at her best in an emergency, and her sometimes careless and blundering habits didn't affect her mental efficiency. Her mind worked rapidly and even while Mrs. Lummis was talking, she was planning a way to circumvent her.

At last the vivacious lady returned to the table, with a murmured excuse for her lengthy absence.

"That's all right," Bumble said, smiling, "and I'm going to ask a similar indulgence. May I telephone, please,—as I've a bothersome dressmaker's engagement that I want to break."

"So sorry," said Mrs. Lummis, looking at her shrewdly, "but the telephone is out of order. The storm, you know. Just as I finished talking, it went dead, and we can't use it till it's fixed."

Helen knew this for an untruth, and a hastily fabricated invention at that. But she saw that Mrs. Lummis was not going to let her use the telephone, and she felt her fears verified that there was some secret work going on.

Mrs. Lummis then began chatting again, apparently forgetful of her impending journey, and as she adroitly led the talk to war matters and around to Captain Farnsworth, Helen grew more and more wary of what she said, and also more and more determined to speak to Patty without delay.

Breakfast finished, they rose, and went back to the bedroom.

Mrs. Lummis sat in a high-backed chair, and Bumble quickly formed her plan.

She drew from her coat pocket a long chiffon veil or scarf, that she carried for cold weather.

"You've been so kind," she said, " I'm going to ask your acceptance of this as a little souvenir. It's a Liberty scarf,—I bought it in London,—but it's been little used."

"Oh, it's lovely," said Mrs. Lummis, admiring the silken fabric.

"Yes, and it's a real Liberty scarf,—to help me to my liberty!"

As Helen spoke, she quickly threw it around Mrs. Lummis' neck and then around the high back of the chair, knotting it tightly.

"You little villain!" cried the victim, "take that off!"

"Not at all," and Bumble pulled the knot tighter. It did not hurt the prisoner, but it made it impossible for her to rise from the heavy, high-backed chair.

Helen quickly tied two or three more strong knots in the long ends, and the firm silk fabric was as secure as a hempen rope would have been.

" Now, I guess that'll hold you!" she said, nodding approval at her work. Then, oblivious to the venomous looks of the captive lady, she took up the telephone and called Patty.

" If you're innocent of any wrong," she said to Mrs. Lummis, as she waited for her response, " you can have no objection to my speaking to my friends. Hello, that you?"

She mentioned no name but recognised Patty's voice.

" You know that little matter you put in the Winthrop?"

" Yes," said Patty, knowing at once Bumble meant the old Governor Winthrop desk.

" Take it out at once,—now,—and put it somewhere else. See?"

" No, I don't see——"

" Well, you don't have to," Bumble was nervously impatient, but kept her voice calm, " only in the name of your country, do as I say!"

" I will."

"Yes; remove that to a place of safety,—absolute safety. Will you?"

"I will, at once."

Patty's clear voice betokened her complete comprehension, and Helen said no more.

Helen drew a sigh of relief as she hung up the receiver.

She looked calmly at Mrs. Lummis. "I suppose you're doing what you consider your duty," she said, "as I am doing mine. There's no use of our quarrelling, is there?"

"I've no desire to quarrel," the speaker was quite evidently holding her temper under control with difficulty, "but I think this a most unkind return for the hospitality I've shown you."

"So do I!" and Helen laughed. "Let's untie the baddy old scarf!"

Still smiling, she untied the hard knots behind the chair, taking her time for it, however.

"I may misjudge you entirely," she went on, slowly, "but sumpum tells me you've used my information to your own—or to some one's advantage."

"In-deed!" said Mrs. Lummis, looking at her curiously, "you're a clever youngster, I see."

A Desperate Situation

" Not so clever as I wish I had been," and Helen freed her captive entirely, and then handed her the scarf, with an elaborate bow.

" As I said, I beg your acceptance of this souvenir of our little visit."

" Thank you, I accept in the spirit it is offered."

" And now, if you please, I'll get off, and you may proceed on your interrupted journey."

" Very well, I'll call a cab for you." Mrs. Lummis sprang toward the telephone with such alacrity, that Bumble intercepted her.

" No, I'll call one. I know the number."

She did so, and her hostess stood waiting, but with a determined expression on her face, that, Helen knew, betokened further planning.

Meantime, Patty, greatly amazed at Bumble's telephone message, was acting upon the instructions.

She took the packet Farnsworth had confided to her care from the old Winthrop desk and thought deeply as to where she should hide it.

She had no idea what danger threatened, but she knew from Helen's voice that it must be something grave, and that the packet *must* be safely concealed.

It was a thick parcel,—an envelope so full of

folded papers that it was too bulky to place between the leaves of a book, which was Patty's first impulse.

She looked thoughtfully about. She mustn't stand holding it! The danger, whatever it was, might come at any minute. Helen's tone commanded instant action.

A photograph album lay on a side table. This was not usually in evidence, but Patty and Helen had brought it from an old storeroom to look at the old-fashioned portraits in it. It was a large volume, holding pictures of "cabinet size."

In response to a sudden inspiration, Patty opened the album and extracted six of the photographs. This left a hollow space quite big enough to admit the insertion of the envelope.

She put it in, clasped the big brass fastenings of the old plush album, and laid it back on the table, with two more books carelessly on top of it.

She heard a ring at the door, and suspecting trouble, she quickly tossed the six pictures she held in a desk drawer, under some old papers. She heard a few words in the hall, and then Jane ushered in a man in khaki uniform.

A Desperate Situation

"Good morning," he said, pleasantly, "Miss Fairfield?"

"Yes," said Patty, with a courteously inquiring glance.

"Sorry to intrude on your time; won't detain you but a minute. I'm Sergeant Colton, and I'm sent by Captain Farnsworth for the packet he left with you for me."

"But Captain Farnsworth left no packet with me for you," Patty returned. Her heart was beating wildly, lest she commit some indiscretion, and she prayed that she might do exactly right in this emergency.

"Of course, not by name." The man spoke low, and glanced about him. "It's a secret mission. But I've credentials and an order."

He drew from his pocket an official-looking document, and showed Patty an order for the envelope left with her.

"This isn't signed by Captain Farnsworth," she said, examining it carefully.

"No; he didn't dare sign it, it's a diplomatic matter. But it is signed, as you see, by Colonel Brent, and it is authoritative."

"It would seem so,"—Patty's voice was calm, though her heart and nerves were in commotion, "but I have no parcel such as you describe."

"Not a parcel,—a packet,—of papers."

"Just what is the difference between a parcel and a packet?"

Patty smiled at him, for a gleam of threatening intent in his eye convinced her it was better to temporise.

"Don't trifle, Miss Fairfield, this is your country's business. I'm sent by the administration authorities for the envelope, and it is your duty to hand it over, otherwise there may be serious consequences—both to and because of you."

"But this order means nothing to me." Patty stared blankly at the signed and stamped document, that was so complicated of wording and vague of intent.

"Good for you! I'm glad you're cautious. Now, listen; Captain Farnsworth said you might be wary about giving it up, and he told me to tell you that he sent you the words 'Apple Blossom' as a talisman. He said if I told you those words, you would know he sent me. I suppose they are code words."

Patty stared at the man. It seemed to her

A Desperate Situation

Bill must have sent him when he gave her such a key word as that!

And yet, Patty was very wary of possible spies or alien influences. Would it not be better to withhold a necessary paper, than to give it wrongfully? Would it not be better to incur Farnsworth's displeasure for not having done his bidding, than to do it if it were not really his? And then she remembered Helen's frantic message. Surely that meant something! Surely it could mean nothing but that the packet must be kept from possible predatory hands!

She determined, rightly or wrongly, she would not believe Farnsworth had sent this man unless she had some more indubitable proof.

She knew that an alien spy in our country's uniform was not an impossibility, and she feared to accept this man's word.

"I'm sorry," she said, "but I must repeat that I have no such packet as you speak of."

The untruth of this did not disturb Patty's conscience, for she knew that aside from the accepted law that all's fair in love and war,— military secrets must be kept inviolate even at the sacrifice of truth.

"I'm sorry," the visitor returned, "that I must disbelieve that. Moreover, I regret to add, I must do my best to find the packet. Captain Farnsworth warned me that you might prove thus obdurate, and that in that case, I must seek the papers for myself. He even went so far as to tell me that they were in the old Winthrop desk. *Now* do you believe in my integrity? "

It was only the triumphant glance of the man's eye that kept Patty from believing him. She reasoned that if he were an honest messenger he would be earnestly anxious but not victoriously glad.

His air of having conquered gave an immediate impression of expected opposition and she was on her guard.

If Farnsworth had really told him the papers were in that old desk he would, she felt sure, have confided it to her, and not have announced it with an air of braggadocio.

" It isn't a question of your integrity," she replied, " but a matter of fact. The papers are not in this old desk."

Colton strode forward and threw the desk open.

" Where are the secret drawers? " he asked, abruptly.

" Here," and Patty showed him the small

hidden springs that opened the concealed spaces so often found in old desks.

With meticulous care, Colton went all over the desk, measuring and calculating, in his endeavour to find the papers. But he at last turned a baffled face to Patty.

She looked pleasantly interested, but said simply, " You are mistaken, you see."

" As to the desk, yes, but I must find the papers. Sorry, Miss Fairfield, but my duty must be done. I believe what I seek is in this room, and I must make search for it. With your permission—or without——"

" Oh, go ahead," Patty laughed, for she deemed it wiser to make no objection, " search all you like. May I stay here, or would you rather be alone."

" Stay, please," and a shrewd glance was thrown toward her.

An indicative glance it was, too,—though it was not meant to be. But Patty's quick wits told her that he wished her to remain, hoping she would by some involuntary glance, disclose the hiding-place.

This gave her new courage, and she determined to look anywhere save toward the old album that held the papers. If he should find them, she would defend them with her life, if need be, she thought. But if they were not discovered the victory was hers. She was convinced now that this was no emissary of Farnsworth's. Had he been, he would have gone back for further instructions, before he made such desperate search.

Moreover, his attitude would have been confidential and persuasive,—not belligerent and domineering.

So she watched him, a little amused smile on her face, that gave no hint of her perturbation of spirit.

She carefully let her eyes follow the directions taken by his own, but never by any chance led him to a fresh field of search.

Frequently he looked up quickly, hoping to catch her gaze straying to the real hiding-place, but Patty was too canny for that.

Once or twice she allowed him to intercept a furtive glance, carefully turned in the wrong direction, and her look of embarrassment led him to turn his attention that way.

But all to no purpose. He looked everywhere, as he supposed, where the packet could have been hidden. He even moved the books on the side table, taking up the album itself, and laying it down again, assuming that the thick packet could not be between the leaves of any book.

And now came Patty's supreme test of nerve and poise.

" I suppose you think you're very smart," he said, irritatedly, " to have hidden the thing so securely."

" It must be so, if that exhaustive search of yours failed to find it," she replied, but not triumphantly at all. " However, you must remember that I assured you I hadn't the papers. You cannot, therefore, expect me to be surprised that you didn't unearth them."

" I salute you, Miss Fairfield, as an exceedingly clever young woman in more ways than one. I cannot tarry longer,——"

" Afraid you'll be caught here? " Patty couldn't resist this fling.

" No; I must report to Captain Farnsworth. He will send some one else, doubtless, who may succeed where I have failed."

" Let us hope so," said Patty, drily.

CHAPTER XVI

THE FLAG AND THE GIRL BACK HOME

Then a rous-ing Hip-Hoo-ray! For our Soldier Boys, and

pluck will win the day for our Sol-dier Boys.

Patty at the piano, sang out the stirring words of the refrain and then began on the second verse:

[252]

The Flag and the Girl Back Home

Our Soldier Boy is a tip-top sort,
   And wherever he may roam,
His colours are unfurled for the freedom of the
     world
   And the smile of a girl back home.
When it's " Forward, March! " he is on the
     job
   With his cheek aglow and his heart athrob;
When it's " Ready, Fire! " with a Hip-hooray!
   He'll fight 'em to a finish for the U. S. A.

Then a rousing Hip-hooray for our Soldier
     Boys
   And pluck will win the day for our Soldier
     Boys,
Off they go to smash the foe,
   And that's just the surest thing you know!
Then sing out a brave " March On! " to our
     Soldier Boys,
   The war will yet be won by our Soldier Boys,
Colours flying for Victory!
   For the Flag and the Girl back home!

Patty wound up with a grand flourish of voice
and piano keys, just as Helen came in.

" Oh, Patty," she cried, " is it all right? "

" Yes, I think so,—I hope so,—but what did

[253]

nappen, Bumble? Who is Sergeant Colton, and what do you mean by your telephone message?"

Half hysterical, Helen told the whole story of her experiences of the night before. She confessed fully and frankly that she had babbled unthinkingly, and that Mrs. Lummis had made use of her revelations.

"Did anybody come here?" she asked, eagerly.

"I should say yes!" Patty returned, but Helen's fear and misery were so poignant, Patty's kind heart wouldn't let her scold the culprit.

"You saved the day by telephoning, Bumble, if you hadn't, there would have been very grave trouble. Now, don't think any more about it; but I'm not going to let you know things after this. You were terribly thoughtless, but I know you must have suffered from remorse and re- gret, so let's not talk any more about it. The papers are safe, so far. I'm sorry it is known that I have them,—but even that isn't positively known. Your Mrs. Lummis is a spy, or, at least, conniving with spies. It was strange you should drift into her house in that way, but spies are everywhere now. Run upstairs, dear, and get your things off, and get calmed down. Don't worry over what you've done, and—listen, Helen, don't tell anybody, not even Nan, about it. You *must* learn to keep your mouth shut. Now, I forgive you, and I'll forget what has happened, if you'll promise never to talk to any one, not even to me, about secret service matters or papers or anything pertaining to Captain Farnsworth's or my connection with affairs of state."

"I will promise, Patty, and you're awful good to me. I was careless and thoughtless, but that woman was so kind and wheedlesome, she got it out of me before I knew it."

"I see just how it was. You don't appreciate or realise the deep responsibility of these secret matters. I do, and so, remember, even you and I must never mention them again."

Helen went off to her room, and Patty turned back to the piano.

It was a habit of hers to sing when perturbed or anxious, and this new song was a favourite with her, and she sang it with a clear, vibrant energy that made the house ring with melody.

" Colours flying for Victory,
    For the Flag and the Girl back home! "

"That's a great little old song!" said a voice behind her, and Patty looked up to see Phil Van Reypen coming into the room.

"Yes, isn't it? I like it best of all the new war songs. There's a fine swing to the music, and a stunning accompaniment. When did you come up from the South? At break of day?"

"Just about. And I'm here only for a few minutes, but I have a warning for you. Be very careful, Patty," Phil drew nearer and lowered his voice, "of anything Farnsworth may trust to you. You remember Herron?"

"Oh, yes."

"He is a spy, or rather, a tool of a spy. In our uniform, among our soldiers, he has been suspected of selling our secrets. That whole performance at the Country Club was a cooked-up job. Munson was the plotter, and he was trying to get from your pocket the letter that he hoped was another and a more important paper. Since then, they have worked silently toward the same end. Beware of Herron, Patty, but don't let him know you suspect him. It is only suspicion so far, nothing has been proved, but he is under strict surveillance."

"Phil," and Patty's heart beat fast, "I would

[256]

defend Bill's confidential matters with my very life. Something has happened,—but I feel it's better not to tell you the details. Tell me this, though. Supposing some one came to me, purporting to be sent by Captain Farnsworth and using as a token of faith a word dear and familiar to Bill and myself. Could that have been learned by an outsider and used, or, would you think it really meant a message from Bill?"

"Distrust it, Patty. These people have almost incredible powers of getting hold of just such arguments or persuasions. Distrust always,— is the best rule toward any stranger. Farnsworth, if he sends you a message at all, by a man who is a stranger to you, will make it so that you can have no possible doubt of its truth."

Patty drew a sigh of relief. "Just what I thought," she said. "But I'm frightened, Philip. I feel so weak, so inexperienced, to defend these secrets. It is a terrible responsibility."

"It is, Patty, of course. But, look at it this way. Whatever Farnsworth asks of you, he feels you are capable of accomplishing. So, make good,—justify his faith in you, by bravely

[257]

accepting the responsibility, and succeeding in the task."

" I can do anything when I feel I'm helping him," said Patty, softly. " Anything to help him along, with

> Colours flying for Victory,
>   For the Flag and the Girl back home ! "

" Of course you can."

Van Reypen's heart contracted as he looked at Patty's lovely face, aglow with love and patriotism. He was slowly but very surely coming round to the opinion that he could never win her heart away from Farnsworth. He had hoped to do this, not in any dishonourable way, but only in confidence of his own devotion, and a hope that Patty's affection for Farnsworth was but a temporary infatuation.

But it was becoming more and more clear to him, that Patty's heart was given once and for all time to his rival, and though deeply disappointed, Phil was man enough not to whine.

Besides, his motto was, " the game's never out till it's played out," and he had not yet abandoned all hope. Also, he was absolutely fair, and never by word or implication said anything to Farnsworth's disparagement or obtruded himself unduly.

" That's what I sing every time I go up in my airplane," he said.   " For the Flag and the Girl back home! "

" I know your Flag,—but who's your girl? "

" You are."

" Nixy! "   Patty laughed in her gay, sweet fashion.   Secure in her single-hearted devotion to Bill, she felt no fear of Philip, and treated him with a serene un-self-consciousness, that went far to convince him of the hopelessness of his suit.

" Oh, yes, you're my girl, even if you aren't My Girl! "

" You mean even if I'm not your only girl. Would you be surprised, Philip, my child, to learn that I know more about Your Girl than you do? "

" Meaning you know more about yourself than I can possibly know about you? "

" No; that isn't what I mean a little bit!   But I won't tell you now, only some time, I will tell you the meaning of my cryptic utterance! "

" Glad to be informed, at your convenience, ma'am."

And then Helen came into the room, and leaving her to entertain Van Reypen, Patty ran away to look after some of her own affairs.

It was that same afternoon that Lieutenant Herron called.

Patty was inclined to refuse to see him, and then thought better of that, for, she argued to herself, perhaps she could learn something from him.

She went down to greet him, with a pleasant smile and a courteous manner.

To her surprise, she found him in a perturbed and nervous state, fidgeting about the room as he awaited her appearance.

"Sit down, won't you?" she invited, but he shook his head.

"I'm here only for a minute, I had to come. Patty," he grasped her two hands in his own, and glanced wildly about, "I'm frantic because of love for you——"

"Lieutenant Herron!" Patty cried, startled by his strange demeanour and trying to release her hands from his burning grasp.

"Don't! don't repulse me! Patty, you little darling, I'm crazy I know,—but I can't help it! I've loved you from the first minute I laid eyes on you! That my case is hopeless, I can't —I won't believe! Oh, have pity on me,——"

The Flag and the Girl Back Home

The man quite broke down, and raising Patty's hands to his lips he covered them with burning kisses.

Patty was not frightened. Often in her life she had experienced the sensation of a sudden and unexpected outbreak such as this, and she was entirely mistress of the situation.

But she was conscious of a strong desire to ask this suspected man a few leading questions as to certain matters, yet it seemed a mean thing to take advantage of his protestations of affection for her.

But, she reflected, all's fair in love and war, and if she could find out something that her Little Billee wanted to know, it surely could not be wrong.

" Please, Lieutenant Herron," she said, at last drawing away her hands; " I know I have only to remind you that you are talking to the affianced wife of another man to make you realise what you are doing. As a soldier and a gentleman you will not, I am sure, continue such avowals. Please, don't, and I will promise to forget what you have just said. Did you come on an errand? "

" Only this. My only errand is to tell you of my love and beg for a ray of hope."

It was not going to be so easy, after all, Patty discovered, but she said, gently, " There is no ray of hope for you, Mr. Herron, and I am sure it is the kindest thing to tell you so at once. I am appreciative of your regard, but I am also exceedingly surprised. I cannot feel that I have given you any encouragement or any reason to think I have an especial interest in you."

" No,—you haven't given me what could be called encouragement, I know, and I suppose I ought to have known better than to fall over head and ears in love with your exquisite face and winning personality. But we cannot rule our hearts always, and the moment I saw you I knew it was all up with me."

The frank, boyish face was pathetic in its utter woe, and Patty felt truly sorry for him.

" I think," she said, smiling, " the best thing to do is to drop this subject right here and now. Indeed I must insist on your doing so if I continue to talk to you. Where are you stationed now? "

" I don't know,—I'm on the jump. I say, Miss Fairfield, I'm all broken up. I guess I'll go away."

" Very well, Mr. Herron. Make up your

mind to forget this little episode and I will do the same. By the way, do you think you played quite fair the day we were at the Country Club? "

" Oh, that. No, I don't. But I was so anxious to be with you, that I took any opportunity that offered."

" Still, you didn't have to lend yourself to—to underhanded proceedings."

" Just what do you mean? "

Herron, Patty saw, was on his guard at once. But so was she. No word, she determined, should be spoken by her that might be misused.

" If you don't know, I don't either," she parried.

" Then we neither of us know, and that's best after all," he returned, gravely. " Now, Miss Fairfield, I'm going—out of your life forever. I've told you my sorry story,—but I hope I'm man enough to accept your dismissal properly. No matter what I've been or done, I'm going to do something for you now. At least, for the man you love,—and that's for you,—isn't it? "

" Yes," breathed Patty, wondering what was coming.

" Well, it's just this. When you see Captain Farnsworth,—don't on any account trust this to writing,—when you see him, alone, tell him to watch out for a certain wire-puller in Washington. Tell him that he's trying to sidetrack him into the Searchlight gang,——"

"Who is the man?"

"I can't speak his name. But tell Captain Farnsworth that it begins with S and ends with s. He'll know."

"If this is straight goods, I'm much obliged to you, Mr. Herron."

"It is. It's gospel truth, and Farnsworth will be glad to know it. Moreover, he'll be greatly surprised. But it will be to him valuable information. When shall you see him?"

"I don't know. I doubt if it is soon."

"Can you telephone—no, don't do that. Do you have a cipher code?"

"No, we don't. But wouldn't a sealed and registered letter do?"

"No; it's unsafe. Try to see him as soon as you can. Now I must go. I suppose I mayn't ask you for anything for a—a keepsake——"

Patty's gentle heart was touched by the sadness in the poor chap's face, and she looked about. On the table lay a little book of verses that she was fond of and had often read.

The Flag and the Girl Back Home

"Take this," she said, kindly. "It's so tiny you can put it in your pocket."

Gratefully he accepted the souvenir, and as he bowed himself out, Patty couldn't help admiring his big manly figure and his military bearing.

She wandered to the piano, and absent-mindedly ran over the chorus of

> "Colours flying for Victory,
>   For the Flag and the Girl back home."

The ringing of the telephone bell brought her to her feet.

"Yes," said a well-loved voice, "it's Your Own. I'll be with you in about twenty minutes. Good-bye."

"My gracious goodness!" exclaimed Patty to herself. "What a sudden one he is, to be sure! He fairly takes my breath away!"

She ran to spread the good news.

"Little Billee's coming!" she cried to Nan and Helen, who were in the sitting-room, waiting to hear the account of Lieutenant Herron's call. But this new information quite eclipsed their interest in Herron.

"Really!" cried Nan. "When? How long will he stay?"

"Dunno. Didn't get any details, only he'll be here in twenty minutes and thank goodness, that other person has departed."

"Herron? What'd he come for, anyway?"

"On an errand," and Patty smiled to think of the ridiculous boy daring to make love to her. "He had a bee in his bonnet,—a most foolish bee, and I had to get it out for him. Oh, my Little Billee's coming! I'm so glad!"

She danced about the room, scarce able to control her impatience for the necessary twenty minutes.

"How can I wait?" she frowned, "seems's if I'd just perfectly fly!"

"Go and sing that favourite song of yours," advised Nan. "That always keeps you contented."

"I do like it, but I'm too happy to sing. I want to dance or fly!"

Patty executed some most intricate and marvellous dancing steps and like a fairy girl indeed, she looked, as with waving arms and graceful gestures, she pirouetted round the room.

"Daughter of the Regiment," she announced, as she fell into martial step and to the accompaniment of the Soldier Boy song, she marched down stairs.

Helen followed.

" Nixy, Bumble, my pet," Patty said; " sorry, but I've just got to see my own Little Billee all alone. So, you'll forgive me if I drop a gentle hint that you're not invited."

" I know that, Patsy; but listen a minute. I just want to say this. If you think better to tell Bill about what I did, you tell him. I'd hate to have him know it, I admit, but if it's right, why, tell him, and I'll take the blame."

" That's a goody girl, Bumble, dear, but I don't believe it will be necessary. Anyway, I'll know that I have your permission to tell and I'll see if I think it's best to do so. Probably I'll think it's better not to tell him, for no real harm was done, you know,—and yet, it may be that I'll think he ought to know all."

" What did Lieutenant Herron want, Patty? "

" Me."

" What *do* you mean? "

" What I say. He actually had the nerve to tell me he admired me. I thought of sending for you and offering you as a substitute. But truly, Bumble, honey, he isn't a reliable citizen.

[267]

He's—well, we won't say it out loud,—but he isn't our sort."

"I know it. I know a lot about him. But did he really dare lift his eyes to you, Patty?"

"He really did. You see a soldier is of necessity a brave man, and it seems Lieutenant Herron is one of the bravest."

"Brave! He's a blind bat, if he thinks you'd look at him twice!"

"Or once even. You see my heart and hands are full with the one man in the world for me, and Mr. Herron's sentiments are not even interesting to me. And now, my dearest cousin, if you'll take your departure, I'll compose myself to await my visitor. Sit still, my fluttering heart!"

CHAPTER XVII

PATTY AND BILL

WATCHING from the window, Patty saw him coming and in a moment the big man had gathered the dainty little figure into his arms.

"Blossom Girl," he whispered, "my own Patty Precious, are you glad to be *here?*"

"Well, I just am!" and Patty drew back to look in his eyes, and then flung her arms round his neck in a burst of joyous gladness. "But you're so high up, Little Billee,—I can't reach."

"Going up!" said Bill, and he swung her from the floor up into his close embrace.

"There!" he said, after a series of kisses, "now, will you be good!"

Patty, laughing and breathless, was deposited on the sofa, and Bill sat down beside her.

"You blessed angel," he said, looking at her as if he could never look his fill, "I wish I could just talk love nonsense to you, instead of telling you what I must."

[269]

"Is it very bad, dear?" and Patty's smile faded at the serious look in her lover's eyes.

"Pretty bad, Patty-Pet, but a soldier's life is not a lazy one. To put it as briefly as possible, I'm ordered to France."

"Bill-lee! Me, too?"

"'Fraid not, Sweetheart, it's a special mission and a hurry call, and all sorts of disagreeable stipulations."

"What are you going for?"

"For my country's good, I hope."

"I mean what are you going to do?"

"Dearest, it would take too long to explain, and you couldn't altogether understand it, anyway, but in a few words, it's to look after some mining operations. You see, my plans for investigating a certain coal mine district in France have been approved by the Powers That Be. It seems that there has been a ghastly destruction of the mines by the enemy and the coal supply for the railroads is imperilled and all sorts of troubles are toward. So re-construction is necessary, if they are to get coal for the Allies' use in the Northeast part of Fair France. My experience in re-building wrecked mines in Colorado counts for a lot, and so I'm picked for duty."

Patty and Bill

"You wonderful man!" and Patty's eyes gleamed with admiration as she looked at the eager, fine face, full of efficiency and enthusiasm. "Oh, and Billee, dear, that reminds me, Lieutenant Herron said to tell you to watch out for a certain wire-puller in Washington——"

"Wait a minute, Patty, can we be overheard?"

"No; but I'll close this door."

"I'll close it, but remember, dear, you must never tell secrets where any servant or any one at all can by chance learn of them."

"All right. Well, Mr. Herron said to watch out for this person, for he is trying to sidetrack you into the Searchlight gang,—whatever that is."

"Herron said this? Did he tell you the name?"

"He said it began with S and ended with s, and that you'd know from that——"

"Whew! Did Herron say that! Why, Patty,—are you sure?"

"Yes, sure; and he said you'd be surprised but you'd be glad of the information."

"I should say so! Why, Patty, you've no idea of the enormous importance of that warning! Him! Well, well!"

" I'm so glad to help you, Billee———"

" How did Herron happen to tell you? "

Patty hesitated. " Well," she said, blush-ingly, " Lieutenant Herron did me the honour to make love to me———"

" What! what do you mean by ' make love '? "

" Nothing! Please don't bite my head off! I only mean he seemed to admire me,—or said he did,—and I sent him flying."

" I should say so! The scoundrel———"

" Oh, come, now, Little Billee, he may be a scoundrel,—I'm told he is one,—but not be-cause he admired me! A cat may look at a king."

" But no cat or king or scrubby little lieutenant may look at my Patty Blossom! "

" Oh, he didn't! The Miss Fairfield he looked at is a very different personage from your Patty Blossom."

" How, different? "

" Well," and Patty sprang up, " this is the lady he saw."

She stood, with a most dignified air, and a coldly courteous expression, looking a little bored, and exceedingly formal.

Then she broke into a happy smile, and hold-ing out her arms in a lovely gesture of welcome came toward Farnsworth, her blue eyes beaming with love and happiness, saying, " and *this* is your Patty Blossom! "

Farnsworth jumped for her in an ecstasy of gladness, and Herron's presumptuous intrusion was forgotten.

" And just when do you go to France? " asked Patty, after a time.

" Dunno. I'm awaiting orders."

" And you'll stay here till you go? " She nestled comfortably in his arms, and smiled up into his loving face.

" Nay, nay, my lady fair. I'm even now on my way to Springfield."

" Springfield! Whatever for? "

" Making some tests for the Government."

" Tests of what? "

" Honey-girl, you can't understand,—but it's a test of the water- or moisture-resisting qualities of certain explosives used in the setting off of blasts——"

" Oh, Little Billee, you'll be blown up! "

" Well, we'll hope not."

" Why can't the people who make the explosives do their own testing? "

" You see, it has to be a Government test,— to decide between various competitors."

" You're not the Government."

" Yes, I am, in so far as they entrust these things to me."

" Oh, Little Billee,—Captain, my Captain, I'm *so* proud of you!   I do believe you're the biggest man in the Service,—and I don't mean physically, now."

" Hardly that, Blossom, but I do have responsibilities."

" Do they wear on you?"

" They do, indeed!   So, for just a few moments I'm going to forget them utterly, and only remember the touch of your pink blossom fingers and the sweetness of your flower-face."

" Dear Big Little Billee!   For such a strong person you are very gentle."

" To you how could I be otherwise?   Now, Pattibelle, what about it?   Can you make our wedding-day an earlier date, and go along with me?"

" You said I couldn't go!"

" You can, if you'll marry me in time.   But I just 'most know you won't."

" Oh, I couldn't, dear.   Why, you may go any day, now."

" Yes, but—can't,—won't you go, too?"

The wistfulness in the earnest face touched

[274]

Patty and Bill

Patty's heart, but she couldn't quite say yes to this question.

"How long do you expect to be over there?"

"I've no idea. It may be for years and it may be forever——"

"What?"

"Oh, I don't mean that literally——"

"You won't be at the front?"

"Oh, no; unless some emergency calls for it."

"Well," and Patty sighed, "I see I'll have to be sensible for us both. In the first place, dear, you'd be hampered with a bride——"

"Hampered! Oh, Patty!"

"You wouldn't,—but your work would. I see it more clearly than you do. All you think of is to get me to go with you. But you don't realise how it would bother you to have me along. Why, I doubt if you'd be allowed to take me, anyway."

"Maybe I wouldn't," and Farnsworth frowned. "But, then, how can I leave you? Oh, my little Posy Face, you don't know yet what you mean to me! And,—after I'm gone, —you'd—Patty! you'd flirt,—you know you would!"

"Oh, no! *no!*" and the big blue eyes were full of mock horror. "Oh, no, I'd take the veil and do nothing but weep until you came back."

"You little rascal,—how you do love to tease me!"

And as a matter of fact, Patty did. Whole-hearted, single-hearted, her love was all Farns-worth's—once and forever, but her gay nature made her love to play on his big, honest sensi-tive heart as on a lute.

"I do," she said, calmly, as she twined her little pink fingers into his big, strong ones, "because you take teasing so beautifully!"

"Scallywag! I think I'll just grab you up and carry you off,—willy-nilly!"

"I never did know what willy-nilly means, and I'd love to find out."

"You'll find out when you're my wife! I ex-pect you to obey my lightest word! I shall be a regular caveman!"

"You're big enough, but you've got about as much of the 'caveman' temperament as a kitten!"

Farnsworth laughed, well knowing that the soft, gentle personality of the girl he loved would never be cowed or coerced by his will. He knew he could persuade her through love, where harsher means would be useless.

[276]

Patty and Bill

Big Bill Farnsworth perfectly understood Patty's nature, and her little inconsistencies and whimsicalities bothered him not a whit.

He was most desirous to take her to France with him, but he knew too, that her common-sense view of that matter was the right one. He knew that, even were he allowed to take a wife with him, there would be many rude experiences, even dangers, which Patty must face, and yet he shrank from the thought of leaving her for an indefinite, perhaps for a very long time.

Farnsworth went on to Springfield with the question still unsettled.

At least, to his satisfaction, Patty declared that it was settled. She bravely accepted the fact of his necessary absence because it was his duty to his country, and Patty was patriotic first, last and all the time.

" Don't you *care?* " asked Helen, curiously; "what are you made of, Patty, that you can let him go? "

Patty's eyes filled with tears.

" I suppose it does look strange to you, Bumble," she said; " but you don't understand, dear. I know Billee would do better work and get along with less care and anxiety without me

than with me. I know I should be a hindrance
and I *daren't* go. I mustn't put a straw in the
way of his splendid career,—I mustn't be the
least mite of a millstone about his neck. It is
because my love for him is so complete, so all-
enveloping,—that I know I *must* sacrifice myself to it—and to him."

"But, Patty, he'll think you don't want to go."

"I know that, Helen. And that I have to
bear, too. If he knew how I want to go,—
how I long to go,—how it seems as if I *must*
go,—he never would go off without me! I
have to bid him good-bye, smilingly,—even
though my heart breaks after he is gone."

"Forgive me, Patty, I did misjudge you.
You are bigger than I am. I should be too
selfish to look at it as you do."

"Perfect love casts out selfishness, Helen,
even as it casts out fear. I know I am right.
I've thought it all out for myself. It is my
duty to stay at home, and to send my Billee
away, with only words of cheer and Godspeed.
It is my duty not to let him know my real feelings,—I mean the depth of sorrow and grief
that I feel at his going. It is my duty to make
it as easy for him to go as I possibly can,—and
that can only be done by a light, even seemingly

careless attitude on my part. I know what I'm talking about, dear, and I know that if he knew what is really in my heart for him,—he would take me with him—or,—stay at home! Oh, I don't dare, Bumble, I don't *dare* let him know!"

Patty's earnestness carried conviction, and Helen saw at last that Patty's sacrifice was because of the greatness of her love, not the lack of it.

"But this is between you and me, Helen. You are to tell no one, not even Nan, that I feel more deeply than I show. If Billee learns of my—oh, Helen,——" Patty burst into agonised tears, "if he should know,—and should coax me to go,—I couldn't refuse him! I'd give in,—and I mustn't, Bumble, I *mustn't!*"

The little hands clenched and the white teeth fairly gritted in the desperation of Patty's resolve.

And Helen at last understood that there is a love that is above consideration of self, and sacrifices personal happiness for the welfare of the loved one.

The date of Farnsworth's trip to France was imminent, yet uncertain, and when Patty re-

ceived an unexpected invitation from a school
friend to make a little visit in Washington, she
accepted gladly. It would give her a chance to
be near Little Billee, and her friend, Rose Barrett, would, she knew, be most kind and sympathetic.

Helen was to go with Patty as far as Wilmington, where she, too, was to visit a friend.

"I shall take you to your friend's very
house!" Patty declared, "or else you'll bring
up in some alien household again!"

"Nonsense," returned Bumble, "I can find
the place by myself."

But Patty insisted, and when the two girls
reached Wilmington, they went together to the
house where Helen was to stay.

Philip Van Reypen was there to greet them,
for he was a friend of Bumble's hostess, and
knew of the girls' coming.

And then, nothing would do, but that Patty
must stay there over night and go to the Aviation Field next morning to see the stunts there.

Quite willing, Patty agreed, and telephoned to
Rose Barrett not to expect her till the follow-
ing day.

The trip to the Aviation Field was full of
novelty and pleasure. Fascinated, Patty

watched the great machines as they swept and swerved and was interested in all the details and wonders of the whole place.

A gay young Lieutenant by the name of Breen was introduced and Patty found him a most pleasant and intelligent guide. With him she went about, seeing things, while Van Reypen escorted Helen.

" Wouldn't you like to go for a little fly, Miss Fairfield? " asked Breen, presently.

" I'd love to," said Patty, her eyes sparkling at the thought, " I'm just crazy to, but I can't, thank you."

" Why not? "

" I promised not to,—promised somebody to whom I always keep my promises."

" Ah, a man? "

" Yes, a man, though I usually keep my promises to women, too."

" A bad promise is better broken than kept," Breen said, laughingly; " come on in,—the air's fine! "

" Fie, fie, Lieutenant, to tempt me to break my promises! I'm ashamed of you! "

" But you'd like to go? "

" If I hadn't promised—yes."

" Oh, all right, I won't tempt you. I know

just how you feel. We all have to keep promises sometimes that we wish we didn't."

The jolly young man continued to keep her interested in the sights and at last he said, " Suppose you just get in here, and see how it seems, I don't mean to fly, you know, but just have the experience of getting in and out again."

Patty consented to this, and took her seat as directed.

Just how it all came about, she never quite knew, but soon she found herself gently rising from the ground.

" We're going! " she exclaimed. " Oh, let me out! "

" Steady! " said Breen, his eyes on his machinery; " don't speak to me. Yes, we're going for a tiny spin, and you can have it out with me afterward."

Patty was aghast, but she realised with her quick common-sense that she must not speak to Breen, or distract his attention in any way.

But she said quietly, " Please put me out as soon as you can."

A light laugh was his reply, and they soared higher.

Finding herself utterly unable to prevent the

trip, and knowing not at all how long it would last or where it would terminate, Patty, with her usual adjustment to circumstances, allowed herself to enjoy it. The day was perfect, the air cold and clear, and the sensation of the strange motion wonderfully exhilarating.

After a short time her tense muscles relaxed a bit, and she breathed more freely. She didn't feel afraid, but felt a strong nervous tension, and an intense desire to get down again. She tried to speak to Breen, in spite of his warning, but the noise of the motor drowned her voice.

She looked about, or tried to, when suddenly she became aware that a strand of her hair had loosened and was caught in something.

Terribly frightened, and feeling sure that to move her head would precipitate some awful disaster, Patty put her wits to work.

Her hair was caught in a piston at the side of the machine, and any gentle movement failed to loosen it. A stronger jerk would tear her hair out by the roots, and Patty wondered if this were not what she ought to do to avert worse disaster.

She bethought herself of a tiny pair of scissors in her little handbag and wondered if she could get them. It was a difficult process, but she managed it at last, only by getting them with one hand and being obliged to drop the bag overboard in the process. It contained money and some small valuables, but all Patty thought of now, was to release her head from that ever increasing pull.

Cautiously she raised her hand, calculating the direction with difficulty.

But she managed to accomplish her aim, and with several short steady clips she severed the strand of hair and liberated her strained head.

Quite unconsciously she clung to the scissors, and though she realised the great danger was over, she felt faint with the reaction.

After what seemed an interminable time, they reached the ground again, having really made a very short flight.

"There, Miss Fairfield," said Lieutenant Breen, gaily, " you've had a fly, and yet you've kept your promise! For you certainly did not go of your own volition! Why,—what's the matter? "

Patty looked at him with such reproach and scorn that the boy,—for he was little more,— was overcome with dismay.

[284]

"How could you?" she stormed, "have you any idea how offended I am?"

"No, ma'am, I haven't!" he said, dumfoundedly; "I—I thought you'd like it."

Suddenly Patty realised that he thought she was a giddy girl who would love the lark as he planned it, and who was only kept from giving consent by a foolish promise. He had no idea her promise was to her a sacred rite, and to break it was her horror. Moreover, he knew nothing of the danger she had been through. When she showed him her clipped lock of hair, he was even more distressed than she.

"Oh, I am so sorry! Can you *ever* forgive me! What pluck! Miss Fairfield, you are a heroine!"

And indeed Patty was. She was praised and exploited and complimented on her bravery and cleverness until she was positively embarrassed.

And the Lieutenant told her that if Captain Farnsworth had any punishment in store for him, he would submit to it without a murmur.

"But," he grinned, "it's something to tell of all my life! Cut off her hair on the fly! Gee whiz!"

CHAPTER XVIII

PATTY'S WEDDING

"AND I went up in an aeroplane," Patty said, looking squarely into Bill's blue eyes.

They stood in the pretty little drawing-room at Rose Barrett's. Farnsworth had just come, hastening to see Patty, on her arrival in Washington.

He held Patty's two hands in his own, and after a deep gaze into the troubled eyes lifted to his, he said:

" Who tricked you into it? "

" Oh, Little Billee, how *did* you know that was the way it happened? "

" Why, it couldn't happen any other way. You promised me you wouldn't, and so you must have been coerced or tricked into it."

" Just what I was! " and Patty described the whole performance.

Farnsworth shuddered as she told of her hair getting caught in the piston, and drew her closely to him.

[286]

Patty's Wedding

"Oh, my darling,—my blessed little girl, how *can* I go off and leave you? In these times nobody is safe from dangers! But you'll *never* even run such a chance again, will you?"

"Of course not. I've had my lesson!"

"And a severe one. Why, the shock might have made you ill."

"It did, nearly. But I had to stay on deck till I could see you, and tell you about it. And then, I didn't have to tell you! You knew yourself! How did you understand so perfectly and so quickly?"

"Patty, you and I are—well, I can't think of the perfect English word. The French would say *en rapport,* the Italians would say *simpatica.* But we are—at one, is perhaps the best phrase. We shall always be so. It's utter trust, you know, and absolute faith in each other. Isn't it, my girl?"

"Yes, dear," and Patty laid her hand caressingly on the khaki-clad shoulder of the big man, as she gave him a smile of perfect confidence. "Oh, my Little Billee, I don't want you to go away from me. I've just begun to realise what losing you will mean to me."

"Perhaps it won't be for long, dearest. Things look a little as if I may make only a short trip, and return soon with my reports."

"Ahem!" said a voice loudly and repeatedly outside the half-closed door. "May I come in?"

"Come along, Rose," laughed Patty. "I'll share my last interview with you!"

"Oh, Captain Farnsworth isn't going right off, is he?"

"No, not today," returned Bill. "But of course, there's no telling how soon it may be."

"I want you tonight for a little party," Rose went on. "I find I can get Lieutenant Van Reypen and Helen Barlow over and I'm asking a few more. I think in these days of unrest we must have a bit of relaxation when we can."

"I'm with you," said Farnsworth, heartily; "I can come, I'm sure, unless something sudden and unexpected turns up. Count on me, Mrs. Barrett. But I must run away now, for I've an immediate appointment."

"Isn't he a darling!" Rose exclaimed, as she and Patty watched the military figure stride down the street.

"Oh, he is! Sometimes I fear I'm not grateful enough for the love and devotion of such a wonderful man!"

[288]

Patty's Wedding

"Naughty girl! 'Down on your knees, and thank Heaven, fasting, for a good man's love,' as Friend Shakespeare puts it. Now, run away and get a beauty-nap, so you'll be chipper to-night. I'm going to have quite a party, I can tell you!"

Rose Barrett's husband was in a position to be informed regarding certain matters, and Rose knew, though Patty didn't, that in all probability Farnsworth would sail the next day for France.

And by way of farewell and also, by way of introducing Patty to some friends, Rose planned rather an elaborate reception.

Helen Barlow came before dinner.

"Oh, Patsy!" she cried, in ecstasy, "I am having the grandest time! War is awful, of course, but somehow everybody who isn't fighting, is so kind, and we've had wonderful experiences. I've been flying twice and I didn't have to cut off my raving tresses, either! What *did* Bill say to scold you for going up?"

"Well, he didn't break off our engagement," Patty returned, smiling. "How's Phil? Is he coming over, tonight?"

"Of course he is,—he goes wherever——" Helen stopped, blushing crimson.

"Goes wherever you do? Of course he does! How you do lead him on!"

"I don't either! He has eyes only for you, Patty Fairfield!"

"Used to have, you mean. But that was before my enchanting cousin came on the scene."

"Rubbish! Philip's crazy about you, still. Your being engaged to Little Billee doesn't prevent that."

"It means nothing to me," declared Patty; "my sweetheart hath my heart and I have his, so, Phil may come and Phil may go, but we go on forever!"

"You're poetic today! I hear Bill sails soon."

"Dunno. That's as may be. Oh, Bumble, don't let's think of it!"

Patty's eyes filled with tears, and Helen regretted her chance allusion.

"Never mind, Pattikins, you must remember what it means to be a soldier's sweetheart, and bid him good-bye, with

' Colours flying for Victory,
    For the Flag and the Girl back home!'

That's the way to look at it!"

[290]

Patty's Wedding

"Yes, that's all very well for you,—you're not the Girl."

"And then, he'll return with colours still flying, to the Girl back home, and then it will be June and the wedding bells will ring, and the birds will sing and the orange bloomers bloom and the khaki on the groom and the veil on Patty-Pat, and I'll wear a posy hat——"

"Oh, Helen, hush!" cried Patty laughing at the foolish chatter as Bumble danced about the room, waving her arms as she sang.

"But, truly, Patsy, you won't have more'n time to get your gewgaws fixed up and your monogramming done, before Bill will be back again, and it will be June. Oh, soon! It will be June! and to this tune,—Tum, tum, te-tum!"

Helen sang the first strains of the wedding march, and Patty ran out of the room laughing, as Rose called her to the telephone.

It was Farnsworth speaking.

"Angel child," he said, "can you leave whatever you're doing and do a little errand for your own true Loved One?"

"*Can* I!" returned Patty. "Your word is my law!"

"Goody girl! Well, then, go with all possible secrecy,—with bated breath and muffled tread, and all that, to my rooms at Mrs. Richards'——"

"What!"

"Even so. Don't faint, but remember you're a soldier's bride,—or will be some day,—and defying conventions go to said rooms on an errand for me. Will you, Patty?"

Bill's tone changed to a serious note, and Patty knew at once it was one of those important matters with which she was sometimes entrusted.

"Of course I will. Tell me exactly what to do."

"Go there, as soon as you can, and tell Mrs. Richards who you are. She will take you to my rooms, and from the top drawer of my chiffonier get a large white envelope,—not the blue one,—that's tucked half under a pile of handkerchiefs. Take it back to Rose's with you, and I'll send there for it. See?"

"Yes, my liege lord, and I fly to obey. Oh, I just love to do such things for you, Billy-Boy!"

"Cut along, then, and don't let the grass grow under your tiny buckled slippers. Bye-bye."

So Patty "cut along," Mrs. Barrett being

more than willing to lend her car, and soon the house was reached.

Mrs. Richards heard Patty's request and at once took her up to Farnsworth's rooms.

"There you are, Miss Fairfield," she said, "there's the chiffonier. Help yourself. My, but there's a lot of secret errand work going on. I don't know how Captain Farnsworth gets into a day's work all he has to do! I should think he'd be worn out, and I rather think he is."

While the lady rattled on, Patty opened the designated drawer and quickly found the envelope in question. About to close the drawer again, her eye was caught by a packet of letters tied with blue ribbon. Struck by the sight of such unofficial-looking documents in Bill's possession, she glanced curiously at the outside one. It had no envelope and in a feminine handwriting she saw the words, "Oh, you dear, splendid big hero, how I do love you!"

Hastily realising what she was doing, she pushed the drawer shut and declared herself ready to go.

"Got what you want?" asked Mrs. Richards, pleasantly. "Sorry Lena isn't home. My daughter, you know. She'd so love to see you, she's just crazy to meet Captain Farnsworth's lady-love. Lena's a bit jealous of you, too! She thinks the Captain's about the most wonderful man on earth! Mind the steps. This hall's a bit dark."

Soon Patty was rolling off toward the Barrett house. Her heart was in a turmoil. What did that packet of blue-tied letters mean? They were no government documents, of that she was sure. They might be cipher letters or code affairs, and really be of military matters after all.

She tried to think this, but circumstantial evidence was too strong. The girlish writing, the words addressed to the big hero, the blue ribbon,—all seemed to say that Bill had had letters from somebody,—and poor Patty fell a victim to the green-eyed monster, and jealousy gnawed at her heartstrings.

The messenger came and Patty gave him the important envelope, feeling a pride in her ability to help, yet still downcast about the blue ribboned packet.

When Farnsworth arrived at the party that night, Patty determined to ask him to explain. She had had half a dozen minds about the matter, first decided to make no mention of it, then concluding she could never be happy again until she had heard his confession or defence. Perhaps some infatuated little goose had written to him,—and, perhaps he had never even answered her. But then, why keep them so carefully and so sentimentally?

In a dainty fluffy white frock, Patty awaited Farnsworth's coming. The party was a large one, but in the Barrett house were many alcoves and nooks where one could hold a tête-à-tête.

And so, it was in one of these that Bill finally found his disconsolate little love.

"Hello, Sweetness," and the familiar voice reached her ears just before Farnsworth strode into view. With a quick glance around, he took her in his arms for a swift, silent kiss.

"Oh, be careful!" breathed Patty. "Some one will see us!"

"Not so; I reconnoitred first. And how is my Posy Blossom?"

"All right,—that is, 'most all right,——" and Patty looked doubtfully at the loving face bending above her own.

"Out with it,—what's the trouble?"

"N-nothing."

"Which, being interpreted, means something

pretty awful! Don't try to fool me, Pattibelle!
Have you been flying again?"

"No;" and then Patty gave a long, steady
look into Farnsworth's blue eyes. What she
saw there was so reassuring, so absolutely all-
powerful to clear away her troubles, that she
laughed outright and said:

"Oh, you dear, splendid old thing, you! I'm
not worthy of you!"

"That, my child, is the one thing I won't
allow you to say, and unless you retract it,
there'll be grave trouble with tumultuous consequences. Do you take it back?"

"I can't——"

"You'd better," and Patty saw from Bill's
smile that unless she did he would indeed bring
about some "tumultuous consequences."

"All right,—I do," she said, hastily, as he
prepared to swoop her into his arms.

"That's not enough. Say, 'I am far too
good for you.'"

"Oh! I *can't!*"

"Say it!"

The commanding officer conquered, and unable to avoid the issue, Patty said, in a meek
little voice, "I'm far too good for you."

"Of course, you are! Now, what's this

other matter, and then we can go out to the party proper. I'm afraid they'll come after us if we don't."

"It's nothing," and Patty faced him squarely, and beamed into his wondering face. "Yes, I mean that. But I'll tell you. I saw a packet of love letters in your chiffonier, and I just want to tell you that I *know* it's all right, and I'm— *n-not* jealous! I am *not!*"

"Oh, you Blossom-faced little goose! Oh, Patty Precious, thank you for dem kind woids! Those letters, as you so sapiently assume, are not of a nature to rouse your jealousy."

And he told her what they were and of Lena's request to leave them there for a time.

"And I forgot all about them," he concluded his tale, "nor would I have expected you to doubt my faithfulness and loyalty if you did see them."

"I didn't," said Patty happily.

"No, you didn't, but it was a narrow squeak!"

But Patty only smiled at him, and they both knew that neither had reason to doubt the other in any way.

The party went off gaily. But though no hint was dropped, somehow there was a feeling in the air as of a farewell occasion, and Patty felt a vague unrest.

But it was the next day before she learned the truth.

In the morning Farnsworth came to the Barrett house and the moment Patty saw him, she knew he had come to say good-bye.

With a white face and trembling lips she met him at the door.

"Come for a walk, will you, dear?" Farnsworth said gently.

She ran for her wraps, and soon they were off by themselves. Unheeding the people in the streets, they wandered far off toward the less crowded areas, and after a time Farnsworth told her that he was to sail that night.

"It's all right," said Patty, bravely struggling to keep back her tears. "I'll be good,—I won't make it harder for you by weeping and wailing and gnashing my teeth,—but, oh, my Little Billee,—I think I shall die!"

"Really, Patty! Do you really care like *that?*"

"Oh, I do! I *do!* I didn't know it myself till just this minute! Captain, my Captain, I *can't* part from you."

[298]

Patty's Wedding

"You needn't, Blossom Bride, you shall go with me!"

Patty looked up in amazement, and saw in Farnsworth's eyes a look she had never seen before. He seemed almost transfigured, the joy fairly radiated from his countenance.

"Patty," he whispered, "the reason I was going without you was because I didn't think you loved me *quite* well enough to go too. Do you?"

They had paused, and stood facing each other, with quickly beating hearts. There were no passers-by, and the sun shone straight down on Patty's face, as she looked up at his question.

She knew all it meant, all it implied, and with a firm voice that had a glorious, triumphant ring in it, she said, "I do, my Heart's Dearest, I *do.*"

"Then——" Farnsworth hesitated.

"Yes, yes," Patty assured him.

"You'll go with me!"

"Yes, to the ends of the earth!"

"Patty!"

"Little Billee!"

And right there, in broad daylight, he clasped

her in his arms and gave her a kiss that sealed
the compact once and for all.

"We must hop around," he said, laughing for
very joy. "Oh, Patty, we must skittle!"

"We will! We can do it. I don't care for
anything but to go with you,—always with you.
Are you sure I *may* go?"

"Oh, yes, I looked out for that."

"What! You expected me to?"

"I hoped, Patty, I only hoped. Now I'll get
you back to Rose's and you and she fix up the
wedding-bells. I'll breeze in about seven with
the minister. Can't get things fixed before that.
Darling! I'm crazy! You *won't* change your
mind—no, I know you won't, my true, my loyal
Patty Blossom!"

There was some scurrying about when Patty
told Rose. That efficient young woman telephoned for caterers, florists and musicians.

She called up friends and invited them. She
gave orders right and left, and harangued
Patty in the meantime.

"Go for a rest first," she said. "Go straight
to your room and lie down. I'll be there in a
few minutes. Helen will help you dress."

And right here for about the first time in her
life Bumble showed efficiency.

Patty's Wedding

"Yes," she said, "I will. Come along, Patty, and take it easy. There's lots of time before seven o'clock, and you've nothing to do but dress. Come along with your old reliable,— your standby, the steady-going Bumble."

Relieved to get away from Rose's fluster and hurry, Patty went with Helen.

"I've got to do it, Bumble," she said, as if by way of apology. "I *can't* stay here and let him go away, so I'm going, too——"

"Sure you are," and Helen nodded, understandingly. "And, oh, by the way, Patty, where's your wedding gown?"

"That's so! Where is it?" and Patty began to look over her frocks in the wardrobe. "This rose-coloured one, I think."

"Nixy; white, if it's only a tub frock! Let's see your white ones. Ah, here we are!" Helen took down a white chiffon, daintily embroidered, and pronounced it the very thing.

Patty dressed at once, saying laughingly that Bill *might* make an even earlier start than now planned.

And just as the bride-to-be completed her toilette, a commotion down stairs announced the arrival of her father and Nan.

"What are *you* doing here?" she cried, in amazement.

"We're here for your wedding, my little girl," said Mr. Fairfield, taking her in his arms.

"But—how did you know? How did you get here so quickly?"

"Ask Bill," said Nan, laughingly; and then others crowded in, and all was bustle and excitement.

At seven, Farnsworth came, looking stunningly handsome in his uniform and with a glow of happiness on his fine, kindly face.

"Are you *sure*, Patty?" he whispered, as he met her in the hall.

"*Sure*, Little Billee," she answered, happily.

"And you don't regret the gorgeous wedding you were planning for June?"

"I like this better," she said, simply.

And indeed, as a wedding, the occasion was all that could be desired.

As if by magic, flowers had bloomed everywhere. Guests in festal garb had arrived, and at last, to the soft strains of some stringed instruments, Patty walked with her father to meet the man to whom she so willingly and gladly entrusted her life's happiness.

Patty's Wedding

Then the guests crowded about with gay greetings and good wishes.

"I shall miss you, Patty," said Phil Van Reypen, his face clouded at the thought.

"Good for you, Philip, do, please! But let me tell you a great secret; something you don't dream of,—yet."

Patty smiled mysteriously, and whispered low, in Philip's ear:

"Your girl is waiting for you. She doesn't know it,—you don't know it,—but *I* do! When I come back from France—I hope everybody will know it!"

Van Reypen looked a little self-conscious, but gaily protested he didn't know what she was talking about.

And then, the time came to go. Like a dream, Patty saw the people all about; saw herself being whisked upstairs and put into a travelling gown; saw Nan and Helen packing things; saw a maze of faces, a whirl of good-byes—and then,—she was alone with Farnsworth in a motor-car—and they were rolling away, as the jubilant orchestra played "For the Flag and the Girl Back Home."

"How *did* Father and Nan get there?" Patty

asked, as she emerged from her husband's first
embrace.

"I sent for 'em. Telephoned early this
morning, and they just made it."

"Early this morning! You hadn't asked me
to go, then!"

"Took a chance."

"Oh, Little Billee! You *knew* I'd go?"

"Yes, My Little Girl, I *knew* you'd go. I
learned yesterday that you loved me—*almost*
enough. So I sent for your people, in case my
hopes proved true, and today you found out
that you couldn't get along without me."

"Well. You are——"

"What?"

"My lord and master, it would seem," and
Patty's lovely face flushed with happiness and
content. Farnsworth drew her close as he
whispered:

"And you are my Patty Bride!"

THE END